P9-AEX-732

STEM CELLS
An Insider's Guide

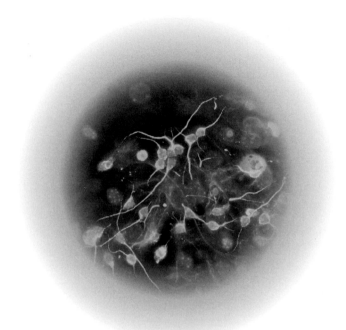

STEM CELLS
An Insider's Guide

Paul Knoepfler

University of California, Davis, USA

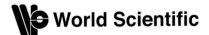 **World Scientific**

NEW JERSEY · LONDON · SINGAPORE · BEIJING · SHANGHAI · HONG KONG · TAIPEI · CHENNAI

Published by

World Scientific Publishing Co. Pte. Ltd.

5 Toh Tuck Link, Singapore 596224

USA office: 27 Warren Street, Suite 401-402, Hackensack, NJ 07601

UK office: 57 Shelton Street, Covent Garden, London WC2H 9HE

British Library Cataloguing-in-Publication Data
A catalogue record for this book is available from the British Library.

STEM CELLS
An Insider's Guide

ISBN 978-981-4508-80-3 (pbk)

Printed by FuIsland Offset Printing (S) Pte Ltd Singapore.

Dedication

This book is dedicated to my family, friends, lab, mentors, and all the patients who are heroes for participating in clinical trials.

Preface

My goal in writing this book is to give you an insider's guide to the stem cell world. My hope is that after reading it you will feel that you are somewhat of a stem cell expert and prepared to navigate the increasingly powerful roles of stem cell technology in our lives.

This book was inspired by the blog[i] I have been writing about stem cells since 2010. Only a few months prior to starting the blog, I was confronting my own mortality in late 2009 with a very serious cancer diagnosis. Around that same time, the one stem cell blog that truly dug into the issues, Nature Magazine's *The Niche*, ended its run due to financial reasons much to the field's disappointment.

At that point, when I was not focusing on whether my prostate cancer might be the end of me, I saw a troubling gap within the world of stem cell social media after the end of *The Niche*. Internet searches at that time for "stem cell blog" largely brought up top hit results ironically consisting almost entirely of websites for opponents of stem cell research and of non-compliant for-profit companies seeking to take advantage of vulnerable patients. There seemed to be no major social media voice for responsible stem cell research and advocacy.

I jumped in and have never looked back despite a wild ride.

I have faced some resistance from colleagues in academia about the blog, but most of the feedback I get is positive even from other professors. These days the blog is the water cooler of the stem cell world; a forum for open discussion. The blog has catalyzed so many positive developments that I feel very fortunate.

---

[i]http://www.ipscell.com

For example, I have spoken with many leaders of the stem cell world and interviewed them for the blog. These people have included pioneers of stem cell research (e.g. Irv Weissman talking about his own mentors[ii] and Arnold Caplan discussing adult stem cells,[iii] just to name two). CEOs of big (and small) companies in the stem cell field have also contributed to or been interviewed for the blog. In addition, I consider myself quite lucky to have talked so often with stem cell patients and advocates.

I have worked to weave the wisdom of all these wonderful people into this book.

Many people should be acknowledged for providing me with great feedback on the book, advice on the blog, and/or helpful discussions on a variety of important topics: Leigh Turner, Meri Firpo, Geoff Lomax, Jeanne Loring, Roman Reed, Keri Kimler, Mary Schneider, Bernie Siegel, Doug Sipp, Kelly Hills, Amy Price, Laurie Macintosh, Beth Roxland, and John Carbona. Thank you! You have made all the difference.

I also want to thank the many people who helped behind the scenes but must remain nameless for a variety of reasons. They know who they are.

My family gave me great suggestions as I was writing as well. I also want to thank my lab here in the Department of Cell Biology & Human Anatomy at UC Davis School of Medicine and in the Institute for Pediatric Regenerative Medicine, a collaborative institution between UC Davis and Shriners Hospital for Children of Northern California.

I did most of the graphics, photos and illustrations for the book myself, but I also want to thank scientific illustrator Taylor Seamount who is an intern in my lab who did four very powerful illustrations for the book as well.

It is important to note that some sections of the book were inspired by my blog posts and a few contain actual sections of my own past blog posts.

I hope that this book not only educates, but also inspires. You have an open invitation to contact me with your questions or comments about the

---

[ii]http://www.ipscell.com/2011/09/irv-weissmans-early-career-and-the-mentors-that-made-the-difference-for-him-in-his-own-words/
[iii]http://www.ipscell.com/2013/03/interview-with-arnold-caplan-part-3-challenges-opportunities-for-clinical-use-of-mscs/

book. I am dedicated to building bridges in the stem cell field, but I tie that objective to both accountability and a never-ending commitment to patient safety. I am very excited to see how stem cells will change our world and invite you to come along for the ride.

Paul Knoepfler, Ph.D.
UC Davis School of Medicine

Contents

Introduction

This book is an insider's guide to the exciting world of stem cells. Cutting-edge stem cell technology is catalyzing a revolution in medicine and may change the very nature of humanity. Stem cells provide real reason for hope for millions of patients and their doctors, but unfortunately they also are the foundation for a great deal of hype, misinformation, and outright fraud.

For example, you should watch the *60 Minutes* exposé broadcasts in the US on stem cell fraud in the last few years and the convictions of the two men from the first show on federal charges.[i] However, most of what is going on in the stem cell world is positive and real, highlighted in a powerful way by stem cell pioneers Shinya Yamanaka and John Gurdon sharing the 2012 Nobel Prize.[ii]

A multitude of intriguing stem cell research is going on right here at UC Davis at our Institute for Regenerative Cures and I am aiming to pass some of this excitement on to you.[iii] Just a few months ago the stem cell field hit quite a milestone as well, reaching a total of 1 million hematopoietic stem cell/bone marrow transplants worldwide.[iv] The number of lives saved just through this type of stem cell medicine is likely to be in the hundreds of thousands.

---

[i]http://www.ipscell.com/2012/09/stem-cell-frauds-morales-and-stowe-plead-guilty-to-federal-charges-whos-next/

[ii]http://www.nytimes.com/2012/10/09/health/research/cloning-and-stem-cell-discoveries-earn-nobel-prize-in-medicine.html?pagewanted=all&_r=0

[iii]http://www.ucdmc.ucdavis.edu/stemcellresearch/

[iv]http://www.hematologytimes.com/p_article.do?id=2979

Even the Vatican is getting involved, hosting meetings on adult stem cells[v] and going so far as to pledge $1 million for a collaborative effort with a stem cell biotech company, NeoStem.[vi]

Through this book, you will learn to navigate the electrifying, but challenging stem cell arena to distinguish hype from hope. There are real possibilities for positively changing lives in amazing ways through new stem cell-based medicines, but there are also dangers. Many people have been helped, while others have already died.

What makes stem cells a life-changing or even a life or death proposition for medicine and society? How promising are stem cell treatments? Together, we will tackle such questions in this book.

It is somewhat frustrating that while there are dozens of books already published on stem cells, these books seem to go from one extreme to another. On the one hand, there are very few stem cell books that are written in a manner that non-scientists can understand. They are too complicated and full of unintelligible jargon. On the other hand, some books are too simple, dumbing down the topic of stem cells for readers to the point that for most people the book is not particularly helpful or engaging. In both cases with the overly complex and simplistic books, another issue is that many times the authors tend to avoid stating opinions or tackling the most pressing issues of the day.

My goal in this book is to find the happy medium where you learn new things and ideas, but are not bewildered or bored. I want to make the most important aspects of the stem cell field understandable to you, the reader, even if you are not a biologist. I believe that you will understand the material in this book, but at the same time you will learn many new things. You will be challenged with novel ideas and perspectives.

You will also find that I tell you what I think. I share my opinions even on the most controversial topics here. I do this not because I am trying to convince you that my ideas are facts (which they are not since they are just opinions), but rather because I believe that a dialogue including ideas and opinions is the most interesting way to learn about stem cells.

---

[v]http://adultstemcellconference.org/
[vi]http://articles.latimes.com/2011/oct/20/business/la-fi-vatican-stem-cells-20111020

By way of background on your author, I have been studying stem cells for about a dozen years and doing research on cells more generally for almost two-dozen years. The focus of my lab's current research is on what makes stem cells tick. What are the molecular machines at work in different kinds of stem cells including adult, pluripotent, and cancer stem cells? How are these cells similar and different? How do cells make decisions about their fates and how can we harness that knowledge to make stem cell treatments safer and more effective? I am very fortunate to have an exceptional team working in my lab[vii] to tackle these and other important stem cell-related questions. I also teach developmental biology to graduate students and histology to medical students. I consider myself one of the luckiest people as I love my job. Every day I am excited and happy to come to work at my lab working with my team studying stem cells and cancer as well as teaching!

One of my other joys is reaching outside the lab by writing a blog that is the most popular blog about stem cells on the globe.[viii] For both the blog and my research, in 2013 I was named one of the top 50 most influential people in the stem cell field in the world.[ix]

The blog is focused on educational outreach on stem cells. It has a wide range of readers: patients, scientists, biotech and big pharma people, students, investors, lawyers, employees of funding agencies such as the National Institute for Health (NIH) and the California stem cell agency (California Institute for Regenerative Medicine (CIRM)), the US Food and Drug Administration (FDA), and everyday people who are interested in stem cells. My hope in this book is to speak to just as broad an audience.

My commitment to stem cells also inspired me to start an annual Knoepfler Blog Stem Cell Person of the Year Award, the first award of its kind. The winner receives not just the honor, but also $1,000 in cash from my own pocket. The first winner was stellar stem cell patient advocate, Roman Reed,[x] who won in 2012 (Figure I.1). It is inspiring

---

[vii]http://chromatin.com/
[viii]http://www.nature.com/news/2011/110727/full/475425a.html
[ix]http://blogs.terrapinn.com/total-biopharma/2013/03/11/top-50-global-stem-cell-influencers-announced/#.UT4qYz9Fyms.twitter
[x]http://romanreedfoundation.com/

already to see the candidates emerging for the prize in 2013. I also set up a new group on LinkedIn, The Stem Cell Group, to which all are welcome to join to discuss stem cells. I encourage you to take a look and consider joining.[xi]

In addition to being a stem cell researcher, as a cancer survivor myself,[xii] I can understand the unique and important perspectives of patients facing life-changing or potentially fatal illnesses.

My background makes me uniquely qualified to take you on an interesting and informative journey into the stem cell world through this book giving you the perspectives of both scientists and patients. Think of me as your own private professor and tour guide.

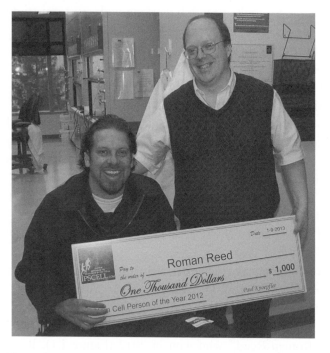

Figure I.1. The author (on the right) giving the Knoepfler Blog Stem Cell Person of the Year Award for 2012 to advocate Roman Reed in the Knoepfler laboratory.

[xi]http://www.linkedin.com/groups?gid=4416703&trk=hb_side_g
[xii]http://www.ipscell.com/2011/01/my-cancer-how-i-became-an-advocate-too/

However, I am not a medical doctor and I want to be clear that no part of this book is intended as medical advice regarding stem cells. If you are a patient or potential patient considering a stem cell procedure, you need to make your own health-related decisions in consultation with your personal doctor.

Whether one believes stem cells will change the world for the better or worse or some interesting combination of both (the latter being my view), you need to know more about them. They are not only changing our world, but also quite literally poised to change the human species forever. My objective in this book is to help you become a stem cell expert familiar with all the key issues. You do not want to be left behind.

On this tour guided by me, your stem cell insider, I answer the most common questions that people have about stem cells and stem cell treatments. I have selected these questions based on years of receiving queries from people interested in stem cells. Some examples of these questions include the following:

What are stem cells?

Why are some types of stem cells controversial?

Can stem cells help my family or me with a serious medical problem such as Alzheimer's or Autism? What about other important diseases?

Are such treatments safe and what are the risks?

How much do they cost?

Why are scientists so excited about these new induced pluripotent stem (iPS) cells?

Can iPS cells replace embryonic stem cells?

Are government regulators really slowing down stem cell therapies? Is there a secret plot against stem cell therapies?

Can stem cells help me look younger or perhaps even make me literally stay young?

What does each of the different kinds of stem cells uniquely have to offer and what are their respective weaknesses?

People interested in stem cells including patients have asked me such insightful questions about stem cells over the years and they have taught

me many things too. Such questions and other equally important ones are
answered here in a manner that the reader can understand, but with solid
science as well. At the same time I have written and illustrated this book
in an approachable way that facilitates a deeper sense of where the stem
cell field has been, where it is now, and where it is going in the future.

Another important question is how stem cell research is funded. In
the US, stem cell research funding comes at a federal level from the NIH,
but also from state agencies such as CIRM. Additional important funding
comes from private, non-profit foundations such as the St. Baldrick's
Foundation[xiii] (Figure I.2) that, for example, funds research in my lab into
cancer stem cells in children's cancers.[xiv]

Battling childhood cancer through research has been an emphasis in
my research throughout my career. I feel so strongly about it that I have
shaved my head for the St. Baldrick's Foundation fundraisers for the last
two years. The head shaving is a way to raise money for children's cancer
research and show solidarity with the pediatric patients who often lose
their hair due to radiation treatment for brain tumors or to chemotherapy.

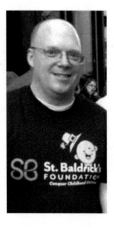

Figure I.2. The author in March 2013 just after having his head shaved at a fundraiser
for the St. Baldrick's Children's Cancer Foundation, which also supports his lab's
research.

[xiii]http://www.stbaldricks.org/
[xiv]http://www.ucdmc.ucdavis.edu/publish/news/cancer/6898

Stem cells are also likely to continue to raise many ethical issues as well that I tackle with you in a later chapter. An emerging very serious concern is the growing number of entrepreneurs who are using stem cells to try to make big bucks selling unproven, stem cell therapies to vulnerable patients. Some even cross the line so blatantly that they can rightly be called stem cell snake oil salesmen, putting the public at risk. Surprisingly, dozens of these clinics operate in the US alone, and hundreds more are selling interventions to thousands of patients around the world, often via so-called "stem cell tourism" where patients travel away from home to get treatments in places that have weaker regulatory oversight.

I also discuss the four main kinds of stem cells: adult, fetal, embryonic and induced pluripotent stem cells (aka iPS cells). Each type of stem cell has clinical promise for specific diseases, but also certain weaknesses. Some stem cells also stir controversy. For example, embryonic stem cells have been at the center of ethical debates for more than a dozen years.

Interestingly, in 2013 the US Supreme Court declined to hear an appeal of a lower court ruling against a long-standing legal challenge to federal funding of embryonic stem cell research in the US. At this point, the lower court ruling is the law of the land in the US and would seem to solidify the role of the US Government in funding embryonic stem cell research, but it is unlikely to be an end to the debates over this area of science in the US. Globally, there remain fierce opponents of embryonic stem cells as well. For example, in Europe some groups are pushing for a personhood kind of law that would ban all embryonic stem cell research in the European Union.[xv]

In this book I will also take readers inside a stem cell lab with an insightful virtual tour. What exactly goes on in a stem cell lab? How is it organized and who works there? How is a stem cell lab able to conduct stem cell research? I also will give you a virtual tour inside of a stem cell itself. I identify and explain for you the key factors that influence the stem cells, how stem cells are programmed by powerful molecular machinery, and what makes each type of stem cell different. In these ways, I will bring you fully up to speed on the cutting-edge rapidly

---

[xv] http://www.digitaljournal.com/article/341453

moving areas of research in the larger field of stem cell science, but without using hard to understand jargon. Where I use technical terminology it is because I feel these terms are important for you to know so I have defined them in a way that is readily understandable.

Beyond medicine, stem cells will also impact society in the future in a number of other ways including possibly changing the way we age. For better or worse, stem cells are also likely even to eventually change how many humans reproduce. Stem cell assisted reproduction technologies that could change people's genetic makeup, once the realm of only science fiction (sci-fi) works such as *Brave New World*, are rapidly becoming closer to being realized and there is every sign that this trend will continue. For example, human cloning and genetically modified human beings may sound like sci-fi, but they could become all too real in the coming decade. Both human cloning and genetic human modification have their strong advocates. Surprisingly, these extreme procedures are technically legal in the US. In fact, the latter has already been proposed to regulators to make human babies that have one father and two genetic mothers.[xvi]

This book also tackles the breathless, fast moving areas of stem cell treatments, including stem cell cosmetics, an area that is now capturing the public's imagination. For example, I recently was a panel member on a live Internet TV show about stem cell facelifts and other cosmetics treatments.[xvii] Important questions remain about stem cell cosmetics. The book cuts through the over-exuberance, answering many essential questions about these cutting edge, but potentially dangerous types of stem cell treatments:

Are these treatments ready for prime time?

Are stem cell facelifts for real?

What about stem cell breast augmentation?

Treatments for baldness?

There is no better illustration of the risks of unlicensed stem cell treatments administered by untrained doctors than the recently reported

---

[xvi] http://www.youtube.com/watch?v=o4K2TxOM-Ss&feature=youtu.be

[xvii] http://live.huffingtonpost.com/r/segment/stem-cell-face-cream-cosmetic-surgery/50d0c006fe344434c100029b

case of a woman who received a stem cell facelift only to have bone grow in her eye. This case was discussed in *Scientific American*, which interviewed me about it:[xviii]

> "Many of us are super excited about stem cells, but at same time we have to be really careful," says Paul Knoepfler, a cell biologist at the University of California, Davis, who regularly blogs about the regulation of stem cell treatments. "These aren't your typical drugs. You can stop taking a pill and the chemicals go away. But if you get stem cells, most likely you will have some of those cells or their effects for the rest of your life. And we simply don't know everything they are going to do."

By the time you are done reading this book, you will be able to navigate every major aspect of the stem cell field. Importantly you will have a strong sense of both the exciting potential of stem cells and the risks that come with the power of stem cells.

Can you imagine the enormous differences in human society and individual human lives before and after the era of antibiotics started? I believe that developments in stem cell research will be just as transforming to our lives and society. I hope that after reading this book you will agree with me and share this excitement. Perhaps you already do.

But only some types of stem cell research are at the point of being translated from the laboratory bench (what we in the lab call the place we do the actual experiments) to the beside. Many others are nonetheless being sold by untrained doctors to patients despite being unlicensed and mostly untested scientifically.

How could stem cells revolutionize medicine in the coming years and decades? The field of medicine, which has relied only on chemical medicines and surgery for thousands of years, now has a third leg to stand on: cellular therapies based on stem cells. Achievements in stem

---

[xviii]http://www.scientificamerican.com/article.cfm?id=stem-cell-cosmetics

cell research that seemed akin to sci-fi only a few years ago are now transcending to the realm of the possible in our lifetimes:

Re-grown limbs.

Made-to-order organ transplants.

Treatments or cures for some of the most terrible diseases such as Parkinson's, heart attacks, spinal cord injuries, strokes, and many others.

Prolonging life.

All of these potential new realities could be catalyzed by stem cell technology in coming years and decades, but there is a catch of course.

We are in the earliest days of this revolution in medicine and not everything is likely to work out as one imagines or hopes. Some things such as the ability of stem cells to potentially be used to "treat" aging remain highly controversial and even if they come to fruition, that reality may not exist for decades. Related to aging, here I propose a new, provocative theory called *The Stem Cell Theory of Aging*. In this theory the number of stem cells we each possess correlates with our biological age and at some point the number of stem cells starts going down directly causing many aspects of aging.

Stem cells are the basis for many very innovative kinds of new medical and health-related procedures. This revolutionary aspect of stem cells brings complicated, ethical issues to the forefront such as how to best balance innovation by doctors and scientists with patient safety. A key question is: What is the proper degree of regulatory oversight for stem cell clinics and therapies?

The central player trying to answer such queries in the US is the FDA, which is tasked with regulating biological types of medicine. A recent federal court ruling supported the FDA's legal role in defining many types of stem cell therapies as drugs and thoroughly vetting the therapies before they are administered to even one patient.[xix] However, for-profit clinics continue to challenge this authority claiming it hampers innovation. I discuss this contentious debate between the two sides. I also provide five key suggestions for improving the FDA.

[xix]http://www.scribd.com/doc/101039859/USA-vs-Regenerative-Sciences-Order-of-Permanent-Injunction

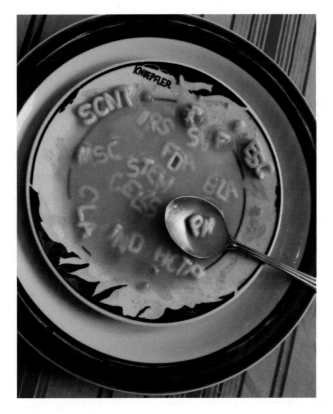

Figure I.3. Stem cell alphabet soup of many of the key acronyms used in the stem cell field.

The overall goal of this book is to bring you up to speed in an entertaining and educational way on all of the most important issues related to stem cells. As a stem cell insider I will answer your questions and give you guided tours without you ever having to set foot in a stem cell laboratory.

When you are done, you will have a thorough understanding of the stem cell field. For example, you will not only know what all of the key acronyms in my stem cell alphabet soup (Figure I.3) mean, but you will also have a deeper understanding of their importance for the stem cell field and potentially for you as the stem cell field evolves.

In the end, you will truly be in the know about stem cells.

Chapter 1

Meet Your Stem Cells

Stem cell technology represents one of the most astonishing new developments in medicine in a century. Treatments based on stem cells have the potential to tackle many of the most troubling diseases and injuries that we might face during our lives. However, our own intrinsic populations of so-called "endogenous" stem cells are vital and need attention as well. They have underappreciated, but huge roles in our everyday health, reproduction, and aging.

As you are reading this you have endogenous stem cells in every part of your body busily working away to maintain your body and as a result your health.

Stem cells in the eyes reading these words.

Stem cells in the hands turning the page.

Stem cells in the stomach digesting your food as you read.

And so forth.

Answers to many of the most critical questions about stem cell medical treatments of today and the future come from studies of these endogenous populations of stem cells that we each already possess. In addition, some of the most essential lessons about stem cells that researchers such as myself have learned come from studies of endogenous stem cells and models developed from them. Therefore, to start this book I will introduce you in this chapter to your stem cells from the perspective of an insider.

The idiosyncrasies, strengths and shortcomings of our own unique cohorts of stem cells are key determinants for how we age and our health along the way. Unfortunately, our stem cells are not perfect. Their limitations point to the reasons why potential stem cell transplants are so significant as a new form of medicine. Stem cells with significant clinical potential include embryonic stem cells, fetal stem cells, adult stem cells, and induced pluripotent stem (iPS) cells. The last is a remarkable new kind of designer stem cell that has nearly all of the properties of embryonic stem cells, but does not require an embryo to make.

What are Stem Cells?

Before we get too far into our discussion of different kinds of stem cells including our own endogenous stem cells, we need to address a fundamental question:

What are stem cells?

I will let you in on a secret. Even stem cell scientists sometimes argue with each other about whether certain cells qualify as "stem cells".

The old saying about a duck that if something walks like a duck and quacks like a duck, it is a duck, does not entirely work when it comes to cells. Appearances can be deceiving.

Cells can "walk" like a stem cell, meaning behave akin to a stem cell, and still not be a stem cell. A cell can also quack or "talk" much like a stem cell (meaning present itself via markers and gene expression as a stem cell) and still not always be a stem cell.

Cells generally speaking are far more difficult to distinguish from each other than most people may realize and the same is true of stem cells specifically. Why? Most cells look almost identical and do not always behave in a manner that immediately tells a scientist or medical doctor that they are a stem cell. Any given stem cell does not have the molecular equivalent of "stem cell" tattooed on its outer membrane. As a result, even scientists are not always entirely sure if specific cells are stem cells or alternatively some other related kind of cell such as progenitor cells. For example, some non-stem cells just have some, but not all the qualities of stem cells.

Time also can be a critical factor.

Cells can change their identities over time. As a result, certain cells can be stem cells one day and then the next not be stem cells any more. It is even formally possible that non-stem cells can revert back to be stem cells later on in their cellular life history. The ability of non-stem cells to be forced by scientists to become stem cells again in vitro in a lab and even in vivo in mice has been beautifully illustrated in the case of iPS cells [1], which garnered a stem cell researcher, Shinya Yamanaka, the Nobel Prize in 2012. iPS cells will be discussed in a great deal more depth later in this book. Whether this phenomenon of a non-stem cell changing back into a stem cell occurs naturally remains unknown. However, the point is that cells, including stem cells, exist in a state with a given identity for only a finite period of time. They are dynamic.

Still, despite the complexities, scientists usually agree on what defines a stem cell. A stem cell has two key properties. First, it possesses "self-renewal", which simply means that it can divide to make more stem cells. Second, a stem cell has "potency" meaning it can differentiate into a variety of other cell types. **A true stem cell has both self-renewal and potency.**

What Do Stem Cells Do?

Our bodies are made up of different building blocks of various sizes. One human body is made of many organs such as the brain, the heart, the liver, and so forth. Each of these parts is made up of tissues, which are relatively smaller. In turn tissues are made of cells. While one can go even smaller to molecules, it is cells that are the smallest well-defined building blocks and functional units of the body.

A very large fraction of our cells are akin to Legos^{TM}. They are structural units that make up the mass of the tissues and organs of the body. In addition, many other cells have more dynamic functions rather than just strictly being building blocks. Certain cells of the heart beat. Brain cells such as neurons work together to make us think. Beta cells of the pancreas make insulin to regulate appropriate blood levels of sugar. Taken all together, the structural and functional cells constitute 99% or more of all the trillions of cells in one human body.

Most of cells within the remaining 1% population are so-called progenitors, which are the immediate source of substitutes for the other 99% should they wear out, be damaged or die. Think of an analogy to a sports team. When a player gets injured on the field, in runs the substitute or "sub". When it comes to cells, that sub is sourced directly or indirectly (via progenitors) from pools of stem cells contained within every tissue.

The body has mechanisms for sensing cell damage or death, which triggers stem and progenitors to proliferate and differentiate into fresh supplies of specialized cells. However, the progenitor cells are limited in what they can do and they also wear out. The ultimate supply source for all cells in our body is stem cells. Through potency and self-renewal, it is stem cells that are responsible for keeping our body healthy and fully-staffed with cells and tissues.

The battalions of endogenous stem cells in our bodies number in the millions for specific tissues, which seems like a big number until you recall that our bodies have trillions of cells. Day-in and day-out, stem cells acting as tiny defense forces achieve things that in the transplant world of stem cells are only a stem cell doctor's dream. In every organ of your body stem cells lay in waiting for the time when you get hurt or sick. Injury or disease is their bugle call. They spring into action and working as a microscopic army of doctors, they pay the ultimate house call inside of our bodies. How these endogenous stem cells function helps us scientists predict how transplanted stem cells, emerging as a new type of medicine, will behave in recipient patients. The hope is that the transplanted stem cells will behave akin to our endogenous stem cells, or perhaps even better and stronger.

The best examples of how stem cells function come from everyday life, even though we do not consciously think of our stem cells routinely helping us. Pull a muscle at the gym? It is your own stem cell "doctors" that fix that. Scrape your elbows and knees after crashing while cycling? Ever wonder how your skin gets better in a matter of days? Most of us do not even give this healing a second thought in terms of how it works even though it is somewhat miraculous. The answer is that your own platoon of skin stem cells mobilizes and acting together as micromechanics they fix you up with new skin at the same time your bike is getting fixed at the shop.

Imagine your surprise if you left your wrecked bike in your garage instead of taking it to the bike shop and a few days later you found that it had fixed itself? That would be amazing, but why then are we not impressed when our body fixes itself?

If you think about it the body's ability to heal itself, which is a stem cell-dependent process, is rather striking. We do not have to think to ourselves "Okay, I better heal myself" and go through in our minds the steps involved, consciously coordinating the process. In fact, we are not capable of doing that. Instead, our stem cells just automatically do it for us because that is what they are programmed to do. In this book we are going to talk a great deal about that stem cell programming.

It is not just injuries that stem cells work to address, but also pathogen-based illnesses as well. Get sick with a virus? Bacteria get under the skin after that bike accident? The only reason you get better is because of stem cells that supply your immune system. Without them, even something as benign as the common cold could prove fatal. When you get sick or injured regardless of where this happens in your body, your stem cells are there to come to the rescue by powering and coordinating the repair of the affected area.

A Stem Cell Fountain of Youth?

Another compelling, potential attribute of our stem cells is that they not only fix disease and injury, they also are thought to constantly fight aging. Together endogenous stem cells constitute a very real, miniature version of *The Fountain of Youth* that we all carry around with us.

Remarkably, without the system of stem cells throughout every part of our bodies, all of us would rapidly age and die within a period of only weeks or months. For example, if I suddenly lost all the stem cells in my body, within months I would have nearly no immune system as almost all of its cells would die as they normally do, but there would be no replacements. Not only would I be helpless against any major pathogen that I might be exposed to, but also everyday bumps and bruises as well as simple things such as a small cut could turn deadly for me.

More broadly, besides resupplying the immune system, stem cells also keep us young by replacing our injured or dying cells with new, young ones throughout the body. This very normal process is called "homeostasis". In the human body it is standard procedure for billions of cells to die and be replaced with new, healthy ones every day. For this reason, your hypothetical stem cell-less author would not only get sick, but also I would age at fast-forward speed. Therefore, if miraculously, illness or injury did not get me, I would quite literally die of old age within a few years or less. The same thing would happen to you if you lost your stem cells.

Sadly, losing one's stem cells is not just a hypothetical event. There are real diseases that foul up our ability to replace stem cells, leading to accelerated aging of the hypothetical kind that I described above. Generally, these rapid aging syndromes are called "Progeria", which comes from the Greek *Progeros* meaning "prematurely old". The suffix "geria" means "old" and is used as a prefix to name the medical specialty "geriatrics", which means care of older patients.

One example of Progeria is a disease called Werner's Syndrome [2], in which children rapidly get old and look like their aged grandparents. While Werner's and other Progeria syndromes are serious, even if rare health problems, they may also teach us a great deal about what we think of as "normal" aging. One possible conclusion that we have already reached is that aging may be in large part the result of faulty stem cells. I theorize that often what happens in Progeria is that stem cells cannot repair their own DNA damage so they age and die quickly. As a result the person who has this syndrome also ages and dies relatively rapidly.

According to the aging theory that I propose in a later chapter, the same kind of thing happens to all of us just relatively much more slowly and gradually than what happens in Progeria patients. But it is still all too fast, as most of us would like to live longer, healthier lives. We end up with a dwindling population of stem cells as we age and I believe that the shrinking stem cell numbers directly contribute to aging. The link between aging and stem cells highlights a key principle put forth in this book: **as our stem cells go so do we.**

If our cells, particularly our stem cells, are unhealthy then we will be too. It is an inescapable equation. The short story "The Curious Case of Benjamin Button" by F. Scott Fitzgerald, more recently made into a movie, has a main character that has a condition that is the opposite of Progeria [3]. He is born old and then gets younger as time goes by until he dies as an infant. While that is fiction, the notion of stalling or even to some degree reversing the aging process via our own endogenous stem cells is at least in principle possible. We may not want to turn back into an infant, but who does not want to be at least somewhat younger? Would anyone not want to slow aging? I call that process of fighting aging, "antigeria".

In addition, who does not want a better quality of life too? A critical factor in attaining these goals is a change in our mindset from accepting "normal" aging to viewing it as to some degree a treatable medical condition. However, despite a proliferation of stem cell-based anti-aging clinics both in the US and around the world, stem cell-based anti-aging is at the present time largely a fictional construct designed to make money.

Today the reality is that even without the misfortune of having a rare aging syndrome, we all start losing our stem cells as we get older. At some point, likely in our thirties or forties for most people, we reach a major turning point of our lives: the stem cell turning point. At that time the number of stem cells that we each have in our bodies begins to slowly but steadily decrease like sand sliding down through an hourglass that has been flipped over.

After the stem cell turning point, as I discuss in detail in Chapter 6 as part of my *Stem Cell Theory of Aging*, the populations of stem cells in our different organs decline each year that we live. There is a direct but inverse correlation of our stem cell populations with how rapidly we age. As stem cells die protecting and maintaining our tissues and organs, after the turning point more and more frequently there are no replacements. This is my definition of "aging". As a result, as we grow older we may get sicker than when we used to when we had more stem cells. Unfortunately, mass IV infusions of stem cells will not counteract such aging and could be dangerous.

We all eventually die. While the official causes listed on our death certificates may be filled in by our doctors with such things as "cancer", "heart disease", "Diabetes", "Alzheimer's", "pneumonia" and so forth, in many cases what should be written in is simply he or she "ran out of stem cells" (Figure 1.1).

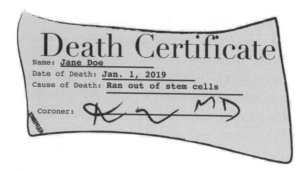

Figure 1.1. What death certificates might look like more often if doctors took into account stem cells.

The Cancer Connection

We just talked about how having too few stem cells can cause aging and in fact it may lead to diseases as well. But even with something as wonderful as stem cells, there also can too much of a good thing. Stem cells can cause cancer and in certain conditions they can make cancer especially hard to cure.

When our stem cells are damaged they can transform into very dangerous cells called "cancer stem cells" that can lead them to form tumors. A cancer stem cell is defined by its unique ability as a single cell to cause an entire new cancer. A cancer stem cell is endowed with many of the powers of stem cells, but is not controlled by normal factors that would direct and reign in these powers. It is like a speeding car with an accelerator but no brake. I write more about cancer stem cells in Chapter 5.

The relationship between stem cells and cancer is particularly significant to me on a number of levels. As a researcher, investigating the similarities and differences between normal stem cells and cancer stem cells is one of my top priorities. At another very personal level this topic resonates with me because I am myself a cancer survivor.

On a day like any other day in November 2009 I was working in my office in my stem and cancer cell laboratory at University of California, Davis School of Medicine. My phone rang and the voice on the other end said I had a serious, potentially deadly form of prostate cancer. Not a "watchful waiting" [4] kind of cancer, but a "I'm going to kill you if you do not do something" kind of cancer. I was only 42 years old. At that moment, my own work and that of hundreds of other labs around the world took on a new meaning for me.

For years I had walked a few blocks from my lab and gone into the UC Davis Comprehensive Cancer Center[i] as a researcher. I had been going to meetings, giving presentations of my work on cancer and stem cells, leading our Center's Cancer Stem Cell Initiative, and thinking about cancer as a researcher. However, one day soon after my diagnosis I walked into that same Cancer Center as a patient and my life was never the same. Therefore, I am writing this book not only as a researcher, but also as a cancer survivor and patient advocate.

I am happy to report that today in 2013 more than three years after my cancer surgery, I am in long-term remission with no sign of cancer. However, I know that the cancer could come back at any time. That possibility is an unpleasant reality, but I have come to grips with it and I believe the whole experience has made me appreciate life more.

I also understand what it means to be a patient facing a serious, potentially terminal illness. Curiosity leads me to ask why I got cancer, especially a type of cancer that usually strikes men in their late 60s. What caused my cancer? Were stem cells involved? I may never know, but I think about it.

The events that collectively lead to cancer can be instructive for the mechanisms that control stem cells as well as their potential clinical use. For example, the same kind of damage that happens to endogenous stem cells over years or even decades, often occurs in the lab to stem cells as they are grown in a dish over a much condensed timeframe of as short as weeks. As stem cells are grown and prepared for transplantation, significant damage sometimes occurs to the genomes (e.g. mutations) of the cells increasing their propensity to act more like cancer cells. Lab-related cell damage to stem cells is one of the most serious roadblocks holding up stem cell transplants from becoming every day tools for doctors.

In contrast to lab-grown stem cells, your own endogenous stem cells are kept inherently far safer, particularly when the potential for damage

---

[i]http://www.ucdmc.ucdavis.edu/cancer/

to them from the outside world is minimized based on one's lifestyle. Endogenous stem cells also are already strictly controlled by other cells and the environment in your own body, which almost always collectively tell stem cells the right thing to do. Finally, unlike stem cell transplants, which can in some circumstances be recognized by your body as foreign and attacked, naturally your own stem cells are rightly seen as friends, not foes.

Stem Cell Therapies

Unfortunately, despite all the powerful things that our own stem cells can do to help keep us healthy and to slow aging, sometimes endogenous stem cells are not up to the task. Perhaps the disease or injury that we face is so severe that our resident stem cells are overwhelmed. Other times our stem cells themselves may be, as discussed above, defective and in that way be a cause, rather than a cure for an illness. Finally, as we age we have fewer stem cells so possibly we just do not have sufficient number to come to the rescue.

It is under these kinds of circumstances that stem cell transplants may fill the gap and be transformative as innovative medicines by restoring our health. As a stem cell researcher myself, I believe that stem cell transplants (also known as *regenerative medicine*[ii]) hold great promise for becoming a more powerful part of medicine and our lives.

When and how might this become a reality? What are the challenges?

In terms of FDA-approved stem cell treatments in the US, bone marrow transplantation (now sometimes adapted and called "hematopoietic stem cell transplantation") for certain blood-related disorders such as leukemia and immune deficiency syndromes is essentially the only option available. **Nonetheless, I am very optimistic that transplantation technology will overcome the hurdles (e.g. safety and immune rejection) that it faces today and in the coming decade. Some of my optimism stems from the remarkable work going on right here at UC Davis at our Institute for Regenerative Cures.**[iii]

[ii]http://report.nih.gov/nihfactsheets/ViewFactSheet.aspx?csid=62
[iii]http://www.ucdmc.ucdavis.edu/stemcellresearch/

In addition we are working feverishly on stem cells in my own laboratory in part supported by a \$2 million grant from the California Institute of Regenerative Medicine (CIRM).[iv]

Scores of other research labs are working in this area as well and there are thousands of stem cell-related clinical trials already ongoing in the US and internationally. The US maintains a database of all clinical trials with a very user-friendly search option by which, for example, one can identify all stem cell-related clinical trials globally.[v] Alternatively, the search engine can focus effectively on stem cell trials for any one specific disease as well.

Stem cell transplantation technology is also vital because there are many diseases for which the problem is not that our endogenous stem cells are overwhelmed, but rather (or in addition) that it is too late for them to fix whatever ails us or the damage is just too great. There are also problems specifically with our stem cells that sometimes get us into health problems in the first place as a result of genetics or random events that damage stem cells. As a result, not only can our stem cells in these situations fail to come to the rescue, but also in some circumstances they are the outright cause of the health problem in the first place. It is hoped that transplants of stem cells grown in the lab may help these problems.

Stem Cell Veterinary Medicine: Helping Our Pets and Animals Too

Of course animals have stem cells too.

Beyond helping people, stem cell therapies also have tremendous potential to help our pets and animals.

UC Davis not only has a program to develop treatments for human patients, but also has a robust Veterinary Regenerative Medicine Program[vi]

[iv]http://www.cirm.ca.gov/our-funding/awards/molecular-mechanisms-governing-hesc-and-ips-cell-self-renewal-and-pluripotency
[v]http://clinicaltrials.gov/ct/search?term=stem+cell&submit=Search
[vi]http://www.vetmed.ucdavis.edu/vmth/regen_med/

led by Dr. Dori Borjesson. Treating injured horses is a big part of the program (Figure 1.2). Here at UC Davis our School of Veterinary Medicine is one of the top in the country (ranked 2nd in 2013[vii]) and just opened a nearly $60 million new research facility.[viii]

Veterinary stem cell and regenerative medicine is an emerging, very promising area. In fact, veterinary regenerative medicine is practiced far more frequently than human regenerative and stem cell-based medicine because of less regulatory oversight.

The regulatory landscape for veterinary regenerative medicine, for example through the FDA, could however be poised to change in the direction of more regulation in the future according to an April 2013 *Nature* article.[ix] Part of the concern is that some veterinarians may be giving stem cell transplants to pets outside the context of evidence-based medicine. For example, the *Nature* piece remarked that some veterinarians are feeling pressure from customers:

> "Many veterinarians offer unproven stem-cell therapies to satisfy demanding customers, says Dori Borjesson, who specializes in veterinary medicine at the University of California, Davis. "Clinicians are sucked into giving treatment" even when there's not research to back up uses, she says."

According to the *Nature* article, just as with human patients, placebo effects can also manifest in veterinary regenerative medicine as well but in the minds and eyes of the owners of animals:

> "And placebo effects — on the owners — can be powerful. "The cat looks like hell to me but the owner says: 'She looks so great. I love stem cells'," says Borjesson."

[vii]http://news.ucdavis.edu/search/news_detail.lasso?id=10542
[viii]http://www.news.ucdavis.edu/search/news_detail.lasso?id=10490
[ix]http://www.nature.com/news/stem-cells-boom-in-vet-clinics-1.12765

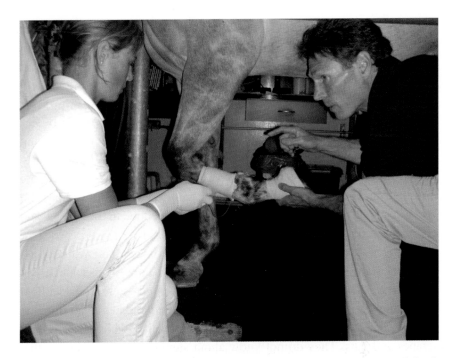

Figure 1.2. Drs. Larry Galuppo DVM, Professor & Chief, Equine Surgery, and Sarah Gray, DVM, resident, treat an equine patient with stem cells. The horse had a lesion on its tendon and was treated with limb perfusion with 10-30 million MSCs.

I would want my dog, Elvis, who I will talk a lot more about later in this book, to have the best care if she got sick or injured. Perhaps in the future such treatments for our pets and animals of various kinds will increasingly involve stem cells, but today I would recommend only having one's pet or animal receive such stem cell-based care based on solid research of the kind going on here at UC Davis. Still, I have little doubt that stem cell-based veterinary medicine is here to stay and will have a growing, positive impact on animals.

Getting Schooled in Stem Cells

Despite the importance of stem cells for our health and their potential to be used as medical treatments, they are only now beginning to be integrated into science educational curricula. While the immune system gets most of the attention for fighting off disease, a process that we all learn about as early as in primary school, our system of stem cells remains relatively mysterious to the general public. As a result, our stem cells continue to be mostly unsung heroes.

Stem cells are the single, most powerful type of cell in our bodies because of their ability to replace almost any type of injured or dying cell, yet almost no one teaches about them in school. Our children carry around millions of endogenous stem cells too, in fact likely even more than their parents do. Puzzlingly, though, with few exceptions almost no one has taught kids about their stem cells in school until college and often not even at that point.

Kids know about red blood cells that carry oxygen and white blood cells that fight off infection. They could pass a quiz on that stuff. But most have no clue about the hematopoietic (blood) stem cells without which they would have no blood cells of any kind and hence no immune system. They do not know about skin stem cells, which repair their scrapes and cuts. They do not know about stem cells in their brains that are building and remodeling their brains, influencing who they are and literally how they think.

As a result, the vast majority of people including adults and even scientists who do not directly study stem cells know relatively little about stem cells and may have trouble with a stem cell quiz. I want to change that and this book is a major part of that effort.

Recommended Stem Cell Resources

#Stemcell social media

There are many useful stem cell resources on the Internet and available via social media. I have learned a great deal myself from them and I highly recommend specific particularly reliable and useful resources. Twitter is becoming more of a stem cell hotbed. If you follow the hashtags #stemcell and #stemcells, you will go a long way to staying up to date on the hottest news in the stem cell world.

I also recommend following some specific Twitter usernames including, in alphabetical order: @CaulfieldTim, @cellstemcell, @cells_nnm, @celltherapy, @CIRMnews, @eurostemcell, @jimtill, @kallosm, @Kaufm020, @leighgturner, @nictitate, @NYSCF, @Prof_ChrisMason, @robertlanza, @spinalcordcure, @StemCellAction, @StemCellTracker, @TedHarada, @TheStemCell, and @ubakaogbogu.

There are also some great LinkedIn Groups on stem cell research. The one I founded is called *The Stem Cell Group*.[x] Part of the reason I suggest it to people is that unlike other stem cell groups on LinkedIn, this one embraces different opinions and strives to be approachable to a wide range of people.

For those with a particular interest in clinical applications of stem cell research, I recommend the top-notch blog[xi] done by Alexey Bersenev. Alexey is the expert in this area and his blog is outstanding. My blog gives out stem cell awards every year and in 2012, I gave Alexey the Blog of the Year Award.[xii] His blog continues in 2013 to be a leader in the stem cell field in social media.

I also am a fan of several other stem cell blogs including the one from the Stem Cell Network out of Canada,[xiii] the one by patient advocate Don C. Reed,[xiv] Leigh Turner's blog that often covers ethical issues in the stem cell field but also other areas,[xv] David Jensen's blog focused on CIRM,[xvi] and the CIRM Research Blog.[xvii] The stem cell investor's website also has a number of great blogs.[xviii]

I also encourage you of course to follow me on Twitter @pknoepfler and you are invited to read and comment on my blog.[xix]

---

[x]http://www.linkedin.com/groups?gid=4416703&trk=hb_side_g

[xi]http://www.stemcellassays.com

[xii]http://www.ipscell.com/2013/01/stem-cell-blog-of-the-year-2012-stemcellassays-com-by-alexey-bersenev/

[xiii]http://www.signalsblog.ca/

[xiv]http://www.stemcellbattles.com/

[xv]http://www.healthintheglobalvillage.com/

[xvi]http://californiastemcellreport.blogspot.com/

[xvii]http://cirmresearch.blogspot.com/

[xviii]http://investorstemcell.com/forum/blogs/

[xix]http://www.ipscell.com

My blog is named after the new type of stem cell, iPS cell, which we will talk about in depth in this book.

Of course not everything you read about stem cells via social media will be accurate so I caution you in that regard. There are many people with agendas or conflicts of interest that make statements on the Internet that are simply false or even intentionally misleading. Still, overall it is important to stay connected and it is simply not possible in the stem cell arena to do so without being plugged into social media.

The top stem cell journals

Patients need to read journal articles on stem cells, but it can be a daunting task. Where does one even start? Stem cells are such a hot topic in science that in the last few years the number of research journals publishing papers focused on stem cells has jumped. Many of the top general journals such as *Nature, Science*, and *Cell* are also more frequently publishing stem cell papers as well. In 2012 I did a blog post outlining the top 10 stem cell journals in the world.[xx]

I am not going to discuss all of these and there is in fact debate over which journals are the best in the stem cell arena. I am going to focus on three journals here. The first journal is *Cell Stem Cell*, which I consider the premier stem cell journal. It has a track record of publishing the most cutting-edge stem cell research. The journal *Stem Cells* is also fantastic and it publishes a larger number of perhaps slightly more diverse articles. A third journal worth noting is called *Regenerative Medicine* (disclosure I am an editorial board member). It publishes more clinically-oriented pieces that have a strong influence on emerging clinical concepts in the stem cell field.

I would also add that some outstanding, very clinically significant stem cell papers do not get published in "top" journals so it is important to keep an open mind.

[xx]http://www.ipscell.com/2012/04/top-10-list-of-best-stem-cell-journals-analysis-and-perspectives/

Patient's guide to research papers: Be skeptical

How should patients or other interested parties read stem cell articles? Let me fill you in on my experience as a guide.

When I was a freshly minted graduate student in my first year of The Molecular Pathology Graduate Program at UC San Diego School of Medicine, I had a still somewhat naïve view of scientific research papers despite having been a technician for a few years earlier. I had gained some level of skepticism from my wiser colleagues in the two labs in which I had worked. However, it would be a few more years and only after more mentoring before I would more fully understand how crucial it is to view published research papers critically.

I am not saying that published papers should be assumed to be entirely bad or wrong, but rather one should read papers with a critical eye because so many publications have flaws or overstate their case. Ironically, in my opinion, the higher the profile of the journal in which a given paper is published, the more likely the paper is to come to at least some wrong conclusions. It is only later or never that such conclusions are corrected. However, low profile journals publish their share of questionable data as well.

In most cases there is no intent by scientists to do anything wrong with papers they publish that are less-than-perfect. Rather, they might be excited by their work and be less able to see its "warts" compared to impartial readers. Alternatively, they might realize the flaws, but are simply doing their best to publish an imperfect story. It is also possible that unintended bias may have crept into the study based on the cells used or the methods employed.

My advice to patients is to be cautious when reading papers on the clinical use of stem cells. Do not believe everything you read and avoid placing too much weight on any one paper. If something is real, it should be reproducible by multiple groups.

A key element of all papers, but especially clinical papers is the "N", which means the number of patients (or samples) used in the study. A higher N usually equates with more power to draw conclusions.

A red flag as you are reading would be statements that seem too broad or too definitive. Mature scientists also usually take the initiative to point out the limitations of their own studies and the unanswered questions remaining so those are good signs of a balanced paper.

These days you can easily find the senior author's email address in papers. I encourage you to email them and very politely ask a few questions. They will not bite. The worst that can happen is that some may not respond, but I predict that about half the time or more you will get a response. This may even pave the way to a longer lasting dialogue.

Be aware but wary of mainstream media articles

It is becoming increasingly common to open up one's daily newspaper and see headlines on stem cells. Findings from stem cell research often are presented in powerful Internet media outlets and even monthly magazines. We also see stem cells being mentioned on TV talk shows and the news quite often. It is not uncommon for these articles or TV pieces to hype specific topics, have misleading headlines, or get the facts wrong. Patients often contact me after reading an article on the Internet or in a newspaper about a specific new "discovery" on stem cells. They might even have seen some stem cell advance that sounds very mind-blowing on TV. After reading this book I believe that you will be well-equipped to judge such media pieces on stem cells. I would also note that there are several media writers who frequently cover stem cell-related issues and consistently have done an exceptional job. These go-to stem cell sources include David Cyranoski of *Nature*,[xxi] John Farrell of *Forbes*,[xxii] Dan Vergano of *USA Today*,[xxiii] Bradley Fikes of the *San Diego Union Tribune*,[xxiv] and Ron Leuty of *San Francisco Business Times*.[xxv]

Try to attend stem cell meetings

Stem cell meetings are a great opportunity for patients to learn and contribute to the dialogue. Yes, you do not have to be a scientist to go to

---

[xxi] http://blogs.nature.com/news/author/David-Cyranoski
[xxii] http://www.forbes.com/sites/johnfarrell/
[xxiii] http://content.usatoday.com/topics/reporter/Dan+Vergano
[xxiv] http://www.utsandiego.com/staff/bradley-fikes/
[xxv] http://www.bizjournals.com/sanfrancisco/bio/3611/Ron+Leuty

most stem cell meetings. I believe the best meeting for patients is the World Stem Cell Summit,[xxvi] which has a powerful mix of science, advocacy, policy, and medicine. Another interesting stem cell conference is The Stem Cell Meeting on the Mesa.[xxvii] This meeting is focused on stem cell science and commercialization, important topics for patients. There are also a growing number of stem cell meetings overall, some of which may be of great interest to patients and others interested in stem cells. I have a helpful online hub[xxviii] of current stem cell meetings that I suggest you check out.

Summary

In this chapter you have met your stem cells and we discussed their defining features. You have also gotten a taste of their power to change medicine and aging, but also the risks and complexities involved. In addition, I went through some helpful resources to stay up to date on the ever-changing stem cell world. As you read on, you will learn even more with an insider's take on the stem cell field.

References

1. Takahashi, KS Yamanaka (2006) Induction of pluripotent stem cells from mouse embryonic and adult fibroblast cultures by defined factors. *Cell.* **126**:4:663-76.
2. Goto, M (2000) Werner's syndrome: from clinics to genetics. *Clinical and experimental rheumatology.* **18**:6:760-6.
3. Maloney, WJ (2009) Hutchinson-Gilford Progeria syndrome: its presentation in F. Scott Fitzgerald's short story 'The Curious Case of Benjamin Button' and its oral manifestations. *Journal of dental research.* **88**:10:873-6.
4. Bill-Axelson, A, et al. (2011) Radical prostatectomy versus watchful waiting in early prostate cancer. *N Engl J Med.* **364**:18:1708-17.

[xxvi]http://www.worldstemcellsummit.com/
[xxvii]http://stemcellmeetingonthemesa.com/
[xxviii]http://www.ipscell.com/stem-cell-meetings-2012-2013/

Chapter 2

The Types of Stem Cells and Their Clinical Potential

Last year your teenage son's kidneys failed, there was no donor, and dialysis was not working. Surprisingly, he not only survived, but today he is alive and well with a bright future when he enters college in the fall.

Your husband had one of those massive "widow-maker" heart attacks last spring, but you are not a widow. In fact, the two of you just came back from a hike.

Your wife has had an apparently progressive form of Multiple Sclerosis for years, but today she is nearly symptom free and her condition is stable.

Your mother was diagnosed with a particularly frightening form of cancer five years ago that does not respond to chemo or radiation. Yet she just got her best golf score ever this past weekend. She and your father are babysitting the grandkids tonight.

How might these possible futures that include hope where there is none today become realities? What is the common thread running through them?

These new possible medical realities and similarly remarkable health-related turnarounds might all be realized through new stem cell-based therapies in coming years or decades. But there are obstacles in our way.

In this chapter I discuss not only the promise of making stem cell-based medicines a reality, but also the roadblocks and outright landmines in our way.

What Stem Cell Treatments Promise

If our endogenous stem cells do such a remarkable job of maintaining and fixing our bodies, as discussed in the previous chapter, why would anyone need a stem cell transplant? Why do a remarkable range of people from patients to scientists to doctors to businesspeople – who do not often all agree – come together on a consensus that stem cell treatments are going to transform medicine?

The answer is that as powerful as our endogenous stem cells can be, they are not perfect. Stem cell treatments show every sign of being able to compensate for the specific weaknesses of our endogenous stem cells and in so doing, look to be an effective new way to treat many existing largely untreatable diseases.

Our endogenous stem cells are not a panacea or based on some kind of magic. For each of us, the nature of our own populations of endogenous stem cells not only says a great deal about overall health, but also more specifically gives us certain strengths and weaknesses as we face injury or disease in our everyday lives. Stem cell treatments may fill in the gaps.

It is also possible that even if we possess the best endogenous stem cells already, at some point in our lives, we may be injured or sick to such an extreme extent that our bodies are unable to repair the damage to a critical organ via endogenous stem cells. Or even if our own stem cells do have the power to fix us, there just is not enough time. As a result we may be disabled or die without some kind of intervention that simply does not exist today. The hope is that stem cell transplants may change that reality in a revolutionary way in the future. Patients, scientists, and doctors are understandably excited about this. Businesses and investors are enthusiastic about the money this new field of medicine may generate for them.

Many diseases and injuries even today in our era of "modern" medicine remain largely untreatable or are refractory to treatment, leaving millions of patients suffering.

Alzheimer's Disease.

Huntington's Disease.

Parkinson's Disease.

Heart Attacks.

Strokes.

Spinal Cord Injury.

Autism.

ALS.

The list goes on and on.

As much as today's medicine is remarkable for treating many diseases, the number of conditions for which current medicine has strikingly little to offer is much more extensive than most of us would hope or imagine. We often do not realize just how many essentially untreatable diseases there are until they affect our lives or those of our loved ones. Unfortunately, our own stem cells that act as our body's team of doctors frequently cannot help us sufficiently for many of these same diseases. Therefore, the hope is that exogenous stem cells used in stem cell treatments of the future will prove effective to treat or even cure these now devastating diseases.

Why might our endogenous stem cells not be up to the task of helping us at times?

There are a number of reasons that I go through below. These reasons point directly to the potential areas for which stem cell therapies may prove particularly useful.

Sometimes the inability of our own stem cells to help us is an issue of quantity. We may simply not have enough stem cells to fix an injury or illness. This stem cell deficiency can occur if we suffer overwhelming tissue damage such as a heart attack. It may also result as we age because in essence we start "running low" on stem cells (more on that link between stem cells and aging in Chapter 6, where I propose a new theory of aging centered on stem cells).

A healthy population of endogenous stem cells for a given tissue might typically numbers in the millions at most. A transplant might use a billion or more stem cells. A thousand times larger army of laboratory grown stem cells, orders of magnitude higher than the natural population even in a healthy, young person, is reasoned to be far more powerful.

The perspective that a billion laboratory-grown stem cells may well be far more effective than a million endogenous cells is logical, but there is an inherent tradeoff that one must keep in mind. In that scenario to get to that magic number of a billion exogenous stem cells for a transplant, our endogenous stem cells must be greatly expanded in a laboratory prior to transplant. The so-called "ex vivo" (outside the body) growth of stem cells raises serious safety concerns. Such problems include non-cancerous but errant tissue growth (e.g. bone in your eye), cancer, and immune problems as well as other issues.

While clinical labs seed such exogenous stem cell cultures with our natural endogenous stem cells at the start, after the cells have multiplied a thousand fold, research suggests that they have lost certain natural features and may have acquired new abnormal characteristics. In short, the billion stem cells grown in a lab from say a starting population of one million endogenous stem cells, may have taken on a not entirely positive, new collective personality. This is an important safety consideration for any potential medical procedure using laboratory-grown stem cells.

At other times, the reason our endogenous stem cells are not up to the task of helping us with an injury or illnesses is their quality. We may have plenty of endogenous stem cells, but perhaps many do not function normally. In fact, the disease itself that we are facing may be caused by problems with our endogenous stem cells themselves. Transplanted healthy stem cells may come from a different person (called an "allogeneic" transplant) in such a case. Hypothetically, the cells could also come from ourselves via an "autologous" or "self-transplant", if scientists could somehow "fix" a defect in the cells or find and purify a healthy subpopulation of stem cells.

In cases such as these, transplanted healthy stem cells are hoped to "step in" and in essence take over the role of endogenous stem cells that are either too few or are not functioning properly. How well reality meets this expectation is the subject of intense study in hundreds of labs and clinical trials around the world right now.

It is also the focus of major debate today as many for-profit clinics claim that such stem cell procedures, which often cost twenty thousand dollars or more each, are already proven to both work and be safe. If you do an Internet search for "stem cell treatment" you will find that quite a number of the results point you to for-profit, unlicensed stem cell clinics that will be all too happy to give you a stem cell experimental procedure if you pay them enough money. However, many scientists and the largest international group of stem cell researchers, the International Society for Stem Cell Research (ISSCR; of which I am a member), counter that we do not have the data yet to make such conclusions in the vast majority of cases [1].

Most of the unlicensed stem cell procedures that are sold today could be dangerous, yet the clinics selling the experimental interventions frequently say there is no risk at all. Sometimes they seek to greatly minimize the risk by repeating the meme that "your drive to my clinic today was more risky than the stem cell procedure you will get here". I believe that such downplaying of risks is unethical.

It is important to keep in mind, though, that thousands of legitimate, ethical clinical trials on stem cell treatments are going on currently too so there is reason for excitement and hope. In my mind, undoubtedly stem cell therapies rigorously backed by science are on the way. We just have to be patient, but I also understand that for many patients their conditions are so severe that they feel they do not have the time to wait. As a result they are willing to consider taking on larger risks. When I talk to them, I generally recommend against it as just too risky.

Getting back to our endogenous stem cells, in some pathological situations, our populations of stem cells may be present in normal numbers and quality, but the cells simply do not have enough time to repair an acute, catastrophic injury before it is either permanent or fatal, such as during a major heart attack, stroke or spinal cord injury.

In most of these types of acute cases, stem cell transplants must be given almost immediately to have a reasonable chance for success. Yet, today hospitals are not equipped to give such emergency stem cell treatments and in fact the FDA has not approved such treatments. I hope that in the coming years, perhaps as short as a decade, this situation will have changed providing a new reality whereby evidence-based stem cell treatments save countless lives at risk from acute injuries that today are often fatal or very destructive to quality of life.

Stem cells are not all created equal. They each have their own potential as the basis for new medicines. In this chapter I go through the different kinds of stem cells, focusing on their relative strengths and weaknesses from a clinical perspective.

The Four Main Kinds of Stem Cells for Treatments

Adult stem cells such as hematopoietic stem cells are powerful from a therapeutic perspective, but they are not the only type of stem cell with substantial medical promise. Today there are four main kinds of stem cells that doctors and researchers are studying to potentially use for stem cell transplants: adult, fetal, embryonic, and induced pluripotent stem (iPS) cells.

Each human stem cell type has its own history as well as its unique potential advantages and disadvantages, which are described as I discuss them below in the historical order in which they were discovered or produced for the first time.

Adult stem cells

Adult stem cells have tremendous promise as the basis for many novel types of medical therapies. There are numerous clinical trials that are far enough along today that within a decade there likely will be a dozen or more new FDA-approved adult stem cell treatments available to patients. Far more will come along after that.

Adult stem cells are the relative "old timers" of the stem cell world. They were the first normal stem cells identified, although there was much earlier speculation that blood cancers originated from stem cells. In the stem cell world, the term "adult stem cells" has commonly been used to refer to all stem cells that are not embryonic in origin, but now with the addition of iPS cells (see below for more) we have a third kind of non-adult stem cells.

What are the types of adult stem cells?

There are many kinds. Adult stem cell types beyond bone marrow-derived hematopoietic stem cells include mesenchymal stem cells or

MSCs, a name coined by stem cell pioneer, Dr. Arnold Caplan [2]. MSCs can be isolated from fat, bone marrow, or placenta. MSCs are the hottest type of adult stem cell today with 306 clinical trials.[i]

I recently interviewed Dr. Caplan for my blog. He pointed out that prior to the 1990s the dogma in the biomedical world was that the adult human only had one type of stem cells, hematopoietic stem cells, so the notion that every adult organ has its own compliment of stem cells back then was somewhat heretical.[ii] Today, however, most stem cell scientists embrace the notion that every organ in an adult person has its own compliment of adult stem cells. Skin has skin stem cells, muscle has muscle stem cells, and the brain has neural stem cells.

It is currently not clear, however, whether all of these kinds of adult stem cells have therapeutic potential. Even if not directly usable for treatments, scientists have found that by learning more about each organ's unique compliment of stem cells they can often discover windows into the causes of diseases of that organ. Based on that knowledge, some scientists and doctors may then even invent possible new treatments.

Adult stem cells are multipotent, meaning they can self-renew to form more of themselves and at least one other type of differentiated cell. A typical adult stem cell can make more adult stem cells and a few other types of differentiated cells. For example, hematopoietic stem cells are adult stem cells that can make all types of blood cells and more of themselves through self-renewal.

Another very promising type of stem cell frequently included in the domain of adult stem cells (even though the name is somewhat of a misnomer since they come from newborns) are so-called "umbilical cord stem cells" or "cord blood stem cells".

Cord blood is isolated from the newborn's placenta and umbilical cord with a syringe and then cryopreserved. This special blood is enriched in stem cells including hematopoietic stem cells. Cord blood

---

[i]http://clinicaltrials.gov/ct2/results?term=mesenchymal+stem+cells+&Search=Search
[ii]http://www.ipscell.com/2013/03/insightful-interview-with-arnold-caplan-part-1-msc-history-nomenclature-properties/

stem cells have substantial multipotency that makes them potentially very powerful for therapies. In addition, these stem cells may have some degree of immunoprivilege (ability to avoid an immune reaction) so they can sometimes be used in an allogeneic setting. A search of the ClinicalTrials.gov website illustrates the potential of these amazing cells as 272 clinical trials are listed among results for a search of "cord blood stem cells".[iii]

Over the years there have been some claims that certain adult stem cells possess pluripotency (the ability to make a very large spectrum of differentiated cell types), but most people in the stem cell field remain highly skeptical about this. To me it seems illogical, for example, that adult breast tissue would (as reported [3]) contain pluripotent stem cells that could make bone, pancreas, brain and so forth. Nature is usually quite logical. The jury is still out on the existence of adult pluripotent stem cells.

Key advantages of adult stem cells: Availability, strong differentiation potential, and relatively good safety profile

One therapeutic advantage of using adult stem cells is that they are very good at differentiating into mature, fully functional cells, whereas the three other types of stem cells discussed below sometimes are prone to differentiating into embryonic or fetal versions of differentiated cells. Such immature, differentiated cells produced from stem cells may not function quite normally when transplanted into adult patients. Another positive attribute of adult stem cells is that they are more readily available and can be harvested from adult tissues. They also have not stirred ethical controversy.

A final, significant advantage of adult stem cells is that they are relatively safer (although not entirely safe) compared to other types of stem cells. For example, adult stem cells are far less likely to cause tumors in transplant patients than the fetal or pluripotent stem cells discussed below. While adult stem cells do sometimes cause autoimmune

---

[iii]http://clinicaltrials.gov/ct2/results?term=cord+blood+stem+cells&Search=Search

problems and have the potential to cause other serious health issues (see 3 papers reviewed here[iv]), the bulk of the literature suggests they have a relatively strong safety profile [4, 5]. They are just not entirely safe by definition. In addition, adult stem cell therapeutic safety is likely to dramatically vary depending on the specific clinic, the treating physician, and the patients involved. The less training that a given doctor has in stem cells, the greater the risk to patients no matter what stem cells are used.

One significant way in which cultured adult stem cells could change that impacts clinical safety is via spontaneous mutation. Every stem cell division in culture increases the odds of mutations occurring in those cells, as they strive to make a perfect copy of the billions of base-pairs of their DNA. While genomic stability varies amongst different types of stem cells, adult stem cells clearly do acquire mutations while cultured. A recent large-scale study found significant rates of substantial chromosomal aberrations (i.e. big mutations) in cultured adult stem cells [6]. Mutations increase the chance that stem cells grown in culture will become immortal, an important first step toward changing into a cancer cell. By contrast, under normal circumstances, adult stem cells are mortal and will only grow for a few weeks in the lab before senescing or dying.

Probability estimates of immortalization events that allow cells to escape senescence are seemingly low and vary among different types of adult stem cells grown in the lab (10^{-4} to $<10^{-9}$ events per cell division) [7]. However, it is unclear in a clinic setting where stem cell cultures may not be grown under optimal conditions (e.g. that avoid confluence, a condition in the lab whereby cells get overcrowded in a dish, sometimes sparking mutations), what the rates of immortalization might be and one can imagine they would be much higher. In addition, if a clinic is growing cultures of stem cells up to 10^9 (a billion) cells, which these days is not unusual, then clinically significant rates of immortalization could occur. Finally, it remains unclear how many immortalized cells in a bulk culture would or would not pose a cancer risk to patients who are recipients of such transplants.

[iv]http://www.ipscell.com/2013/02/three-papers-from-2012-that-raise-serious-safety-concerns-about-autologous-stem-cell-treatments/

These complex issues necessitate regulatory oversight for amplified cell products including adult stem cells. It is the responsibility of those intending to transplant stem cells into customers to prove that the cells are safe before they inject even one person. However, usually dubious clinics just starting treating patients with an adult stem cell product that has an unknown safety profile. Paradoxically most of the time the clinics and their advocates challenge scientists to prove the cells are unsafe, before they will supposedly stop treating patients.

Key potential weaknesses of adult stem cells: Limited potential and engraftment

One relative weakness of adult stem cells is their limited potency. For example, adult stem cells derived from muscle do not, without significant artificial intervention from researchers, readily make brain cells or other kinds of specialized cells beyond muscle.

Another issue is that there is little evidence that transplanted adult stem cells significantly engraft (meaning integrate stably into host tissues) in patients. Transplanted stem cells also do not tend to fare well in patients who have existing autoimmune diseases with persistently hyperactive immune systems that may kill transplants.

There are currently hundreds of clinic trials using adult stem cells around the world for almost every imaginable disease or injury. In addition, adult stem cells are the basis of the vast majority of unlicensed, for-profit stem cell experimental therapies being sold globally. Therefore, as is true with many things in the stem cell arena, there are both positives and negatives associated with adult stem cells.

Another issue with adult stem cells is that so many relatively untrained people are using them as the basis for clinical therapies. Dr. Caplan, the MSC pioneer had a great quote for my blog that resonates here: "All MSCs are good if no one screwed them up!"[v]

---

[v]http://www.ipscell.com/2013/03/interview-with-arnold-caplan-part-3-challenges-opportunities-for-clinical-use-of-mscs/

Fetal stem cells

Fetal stem cells are also sometimes mistakenly referred to as "adult" stem cells, since they are not embryonic in origin. Recall that a fetus is at a much later stage in human development than an embryo, but is not an adult by any stretch of the imagination. Fetuses have organs including brains, hearts, etc. Embryos can have as few as one single cell and do not necessarily have a brain or other organs yet.

Key advantages versus disadvantages of fetal stem cells: Potency versus ethical controversy

Unlike embryonic stem cells, which are produced from early stage blastocyst embryos leftover from in vitro fertilization (IVF) procedures and have nothing to do with abortions since they were never part of pregnancies (see more below), fetal stem cells are exclusively produced from abortions. This is a very critical distinction. Despite this reality, interestingly, fetal stem cells have not generated anywhere near the same level of attention and opposition by pro-life activists, who so vocally oppose embryonic stem cells. The reasons why this is so remain unclear.

Fetal stem cells have some of the advantages of embryonic stem cells including a greater potency than adult stem cells, however fetal stem cells are not pluripotent. Fetal stem cells also tend to be more highly proliferative than adult stem cells. This can be both a positive characteristic as they can quickly grow tissues containing multiple different cell types (e.g. in a culture dish as seen with mouse fetal neural stem cells in Figure 2.1) as well as a disadvantage as they appear to have higher potential to cause cancer or lead to tissue damage in a transplant recipient through out-of-control abnormal tissue growth. This greater inherent propensity to cause tumors makes sense when you consider that the natural job of fetal stem cells is to grow whole tissues or organs in a rapid fashion during development. The explosive organ growth mediated by fetal stem cells normally during human development has some parallels to tumor growth.

Currently there are a number of clinical trials based on fetal neural stem cells, but far fewer than with adult stem cells.

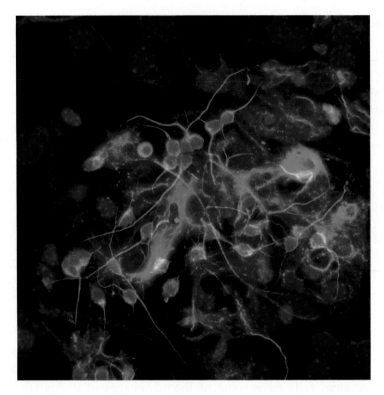

Figure 2.1. A photo I took on the microscope of fetal mouse neural stem cells differentiated into neurons (red) and glia (green). Nuclei are stained blue with a DNA stain called DAPI (4',6-diamidino-2-phenylindole).

Embryonic stem cells

Embryonic stem cells are an unusual type of stem cell derived from an early stage of embryo called a blastocyst that is formed only a few days after fertilization in a dish during IVF procedures. Certain cells of the blastocyst are termed "pluripotent", meaning they can make every type of cell in the human body, but not of the placenta. The same pluripotency is an attribute of embryonic stem cells too.

Embryonic stem cells are small round cells that grow in compact colonies on so-called "feeder cells" that support the embryonic stem cells by secreting cellular growth and survival factors (Figure 2.2).

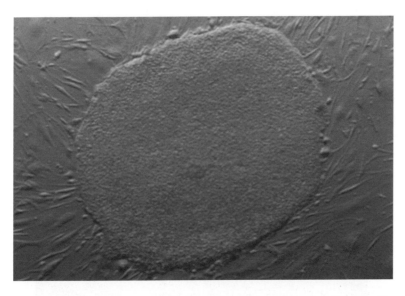

Figure 2.2. Photomicrograph of H1 human embryonic stem cell colony (round object in the middle consisting of hundreds or thousands of small cells packed together) growing on top of spindle-shaped mouse embryonic fibroblast feeder layer cells (for more on feeder cells see Chapter 5). 6X magnification. Image credit, Knoepfler lab, Dr. Bonnie Barrilleaux.

A short primer of human embryonic development is in order. After a sperm successful fertilizes a human oocyte, that fertilized egg is called a zygote. A growth program kicks into gear inside this one-celled embryo and soon it divides into two cells. Then each of the two cells divides making a four-celled embryo collectively. This doubling process continues such that roughly each cell continues to divide (although not in perfect synchrony), doubling the total number of cells every day or so.

In human development, when this doubling process yields an embryo with about one hundred cells, it forms a fluid-filled space in the middle called a blastocoel and the embryo is called a "blastocyst". The embryo also has a special structure called the inner cell mass (ICM; Figure 2.3). These exact same events occur in a dish in a laboratory incubator during IVF procedures.

The cells of the ICM together form the part of the blastocyst that will, assuming the embryo is healthy and successfully implants in a womb, ultimately form the actual organism whether it is a mouse, human, rhino, or a host of other animals. The rest of the blastocyst cells form what are called "extraembryonic tissues" such as the placenta.

The cells of the ICM have pluripotency since they need to ultimately generate the full spectrum of hundreds of differentiated cell types in a whole organism. In turn when blastocysts left over from IVF are cultured to establish embryonic stem cell lines, such lines arise from cells of the ICM.

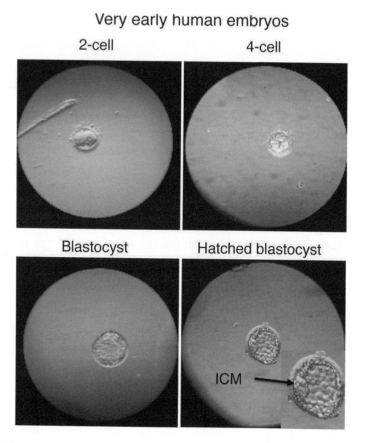

Figure 2.3. Photomicrograph of early human embryo development. An arrow in the inset higher magnification view of the hatched blastocyst (breaking out of the zona pellucida) indicates the inner cell mass (ICM) that can produce embryonic stem cells when cultured. Photos courtesy of Meri Firpo.

I want to stress that embryonic stem cells, despite their similarities to and origin from the ICM cells, do not exist naturally in embryos, but are a laboratory creation. Embryonic stem cells were first propagated from mice by a number of groups (interestingly using knowledge from cancer studies, more on that in later chapters) including Gail Martin [8] and Martin Evans [9]. It was almost two decades later that James Thomson first propagated human embryonic stem cells [10].

Key advantage of embryonic stem cells: Pluripotency

Why do we need embryonic stem cells?

The main advantage and unique attribute of embryonic stem cells is their pluripotency. In principle they can form every type of human cell that resides in the actual human body meaning that they in theory could be used to address a very wide range of human diseases.

Embryonic stem cells, because of their pluripotency, can also grow to form actual tissues and organs, something adult stem cells generally are incapable of doing. In theory iPS cells can do the same kinds of things as embryonic stem cells, but the safety of iPS cell-based treatments is not clear at this time and there are unique reasons (see more on that in the iPS cell section below) for concern about iPS cell safety.

Key disadvantages of embryonic stem cells I: Ethical controversy

Ethical concerns surrounding the study and use of human embryonic stem cells arise for some people because of the question of when human life begins. My view is that there is no one "right" answer as to when human life begins. Notable possibilities (discussed in more depth in Chapter 12) include the following: at conception, at implantation, when the heart starts beating, when distinctive human brain activity arises, when the fetus can survive outside the womb, and at birth. Opponents of embryonic stem cell research generally make the case that human life begins at conception so that deriving embryonic stem cell lines a few days later from leftover IVF blastocysts, from their perspective, destroys a human life.

My own view is that a living human being only begins to exist much later than conception and even later than the blastocyst stage of human development from which embryonic stem cells are derived (more on the ethical issues invoked in this area in Chapter 12). I have not, however, decided for myself at what later point we can call the developing fetus a real human being. I also respect other viewpoints on this question.

It is notable that in the debate surrounding human embryonic stem cells that such cells are not ever derived from pregnancies, but rather from cryogenically preserved human blastocysts leftover from IVF procedures. In most polls I have seen, a majority of people in the US and in many countries around the world supports the use of leftover IVF embryos for embryonic stem cell research rather than have the embryos be discarded as biohazardous waste, but there is also opposition.

The only other even hypothetical source of embryonic stem cells is from a method called somatic cell nuclear transfer (SCNT), a process that to my knowledge has only once successfully been achieved in a genetically normal form in humans. During SCNT as conducted in other species such as mice or sheep, the nucleus of a somatic cell (a non- stem cell) is swapped for the nucleus of an oocyte, which can then lead to production of embryonic stem cells or to a low rate of mostly normal development and ultimately a fully mature animal, at least in some lower organisms.

The first example of such SCNT-based cloning was the sheep Dolly (more on Dolly and human cloning in Chapter 12). However, successful human SCNT has only been reported by one laboratory. One other publication reported producing a genetically abnormal human embryonic stem cell line that contained three instead of the normal two copies of chromosomes [11]. Even for sheep such as Dolly and for other cloned mammals such as cows, it is thought that the process results in a significant rate of abnormalities, sometimes not evident until the animal is maturing.

The ethical debate over embryonic stem cells has also has entered the courts in the US. Federal funding of embryonic stem cell research was challenged in terms of its legality. Notably, a federal court ruling in 2012 established the legality of funding of embryonic stem cell research. In 2013 the US Supreme Court declined to hear an appeal of the case, meaning that opponents of such research suffered a major blow and it is difficult to see them mounting a new successful challenge at the legal level in the US [12]. However, in Europe, a recent ruling that embryonic stem cell research could not be patented has kept the debate more lively there [13].

It is also worth noting that the status of federal funding of embryonic stem cell research was in doubt for many years in the US. While President George W. Bush allowed federal funding of research on a very limited number of old embryonic stem cell lines, he restricted the research greatly overall. During the Bush years, the federal approach to embryonic stem cell research and its funding were relatively hostile.

In part to address this problem, some inspired leaders including Robert Klein created Proposition 71 (aka Prop. 71) in California that led to the creation of CIRM,[vi] the California stem cell agency. Almost two-dozen Nobel Laureates as well some key Republicans including then California Governor Arnold Schwarzenegger supported Prop. 71 and the creation of CIRM.

Prop. 71 was passed in 2004 with a remarkable 59% of the vote. Two great father-son patient advocates, Don C. Reed and Roman Reed, played key roles in making Prop. 71 and CIRM a reality. I believe that the creation of CIRM was a watershed moment in the history of the stem cell field not just in America, but also more globally.

Since that time, the climate for embryonic stem cell research has improved substantially as discussed above. However, one has to keep in the mind the more challenging climate back in 2004 to appreciate just how revolutionary CIRM was at that time. Prop. 71 had some powerful opposition including the Roman Catholic Church, some fiscal conservatives, and formidable Republican politicians.

Nonetheless, Californians wisely supported creation of CIRM, which has not only improved the California economy, but also led the way in the stem cell field well beyond embryonic stem cell research. In addition, the creation of CIRM has inspired the formation of many other state and national stem cell agencies that are doing wonderful work. Taken together, the opposition to embryonic stem cell research and the creation of CIRM provide the lesson that sometimes challenges can be opportunities for positive, even transformative change for good.

[vi]http://www.cirm.ca.gov/about-cirm/our-history

Key disadvantages of embryonic stem cells II: Immune issues

Another potential challenge in using embryonic stem cells for transplantation therapies is that they will be by definition allogeneic (not self), meaning cells are transplanted into a patient that are not genetically identical to that patient. Embryonic stem cell therapies will always be allogeneic unless researchers in the future can find a way to create embryonic stem cell lines from specific human patients using SCNT or other technology.

By contrast, autologous transplants are matched such that a person's own cells are given back to them. The challenge with allogeneic therapies such as those based on human embryonic stem cells is that the recipient's immune system may recognize the cells as foreign, attack and kill them. Most embryonic stem cell-based treatments will require immunosuppression of the kind given to organ transplant recipients. This is not a deal breaker issue, however, as transient immunosuppression appears effective in early clinical trials by the company Advanced Cell Technology (ACT) for their human embryonic stem cell-based therapy for macular degeneration, the leading cause of blindness.

There is still debate as to whether stem cells and their differentiated progeny might possess some degree of a characteristic called "immunoprivilege", a stealthiness that allows cells to evade much of the immune system response even in an allogeneic context. The question of whether embryonic stem cells and perhaps other stem cells are truly immunoprivileged remains open.

Key disadvantages of embryonic stem cells III: Teratoma formation and safety

Another concern about clinical use of embryonic stem cell-based therapies is that these cells have the ability to form an unusual tumor called a "teratoma". The name teratoma literally means "monster tumor", and there is good reason for that nomenclature. These tumors look monstrous when observed by eye, akin to an animal put into a developmental blender. However, histological images of teratoma can be quite striking and some consider them beautiful (Figure 2.4). Teratomas, unlike almost any other kind of tumor, are inherently very heterogeneous. They contain a host of differentiated tissues mixed together in a developmental jumble due to the pluripotency of the cells that drive the growth of the tumor.

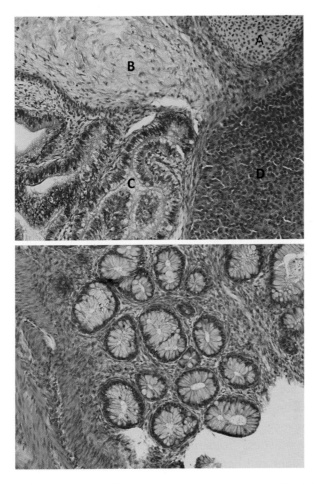

Figure 2.4. Histological sections of experimental human teratomas. (Top) Presumptive tissue types: A = cartilage, B = connective/adipose tissue, C = mucous glands, and D = mature brain. (Bottom) Teratoma including secretory glands. Teratomas shown were produced from human iPS cells, but teratomas produced from embryonic stem cells are similar. These are sections of teratoma stained with the general histological dye combination called hematoxylin and eosin. Image Credit, Knoepfler Lab, Dr. Bonnie Barrilleaux.

It is theorized that a naturally occurring teratoma arises from leftover pluripotent stem cells that somehow never differentiated during human development. These developmental carryovers eventually go awry in children or more rarely in adults, "thinking" (i.e. being programmed autonomously) that they are still in an embryo and their job is to build an embryo. But of course, the context for this embryonic type of growth is absent in a child or adult, so things go very wrong.

As a result, teratomas usually contain a panoply of tissues that can include skin, cartilage, bone, hair, sweat glands, brain, and so forth. Therefore, when the first teratomas were removed from patients (or the deceased) and examined, those doing the primitive surgery were shocked to find the mess inside and called it the "monster tumor". Their reaction is not surprising given that a teratoma may have body odor, a mess of hair, part an eye staring out at you, and teeth.

Teratomas are not just spontaneous tumors that occur in people and other animals, but they are also intentionally produced in research labs studying pluripotent stem cells. If one injects embryonic stem cells under the skin of immunodeficient mice, for example, often times the stem cells will form teratoma tumors. In fact, this approach is used as a test of the pluripotency of stem cells. Pluripotency can also be assessed without using mice via another method call "embryoid body formation" in which stem cells are aggregated together and allowed to differentiate in culture as a floating mass.

In the laboratory context, paradoxically scientists almost always view teratoma formation by stem cells as a good thing since it means the cells in question are pluripotent. However, from a clinical perspective, the teratoma-forming activity represents one of the most serious roadblocks to translating embryonic stem cell therapies to the clinic.

In a hypothetical scenario of treating an injured heart with an embryonic stem cell-based therapy, we might successfully repair the heart, but if the cells used also cause a few 1-gram teratoma tumors to form in the heart as a side effect, the patient is likely going to die. The same kind of negative outcome could occur via teratoma formation in almost any tissue receiving an embryonic stem cell-based transplant. For example, imagine a dozen tumors the size of grapes forming inside a person's spine, brain, liver, or any other organ that received an

embryonic stem cell-based treatment. The organ could easily be functionally destroyed and the patient severally injured or killed.

As a result, most biomedical scientists and doctors imagine using embryonic stem cells for therapies only indirectly. They first pre-differentiate the embryonic stem cells into specific cells/tissues that lack the ability to cause teratoma. In this scenario, a future embryonic stem cell-based therapy for a heart attack would be based not on direct transplant of embryonic stem cells themselves, but rather of heart cells produced from the embryonic stem cells. For such a therapy, the goal would be to have no residual undifferentiated embryonic stem cells.

Advanced Cell Technology (ACT) is conducting FDA-approved clinical trials using retinal pigmented epithelial (RPE) cells made from embryonic stem cells. During the process to make RPEs, ACT goes to great lengths to make sure that nearly zero residual embryonic stem cells are present with the RPEs during the transplant into the eye. The RPE transplant has the objective of replacing endogenous RPEs that die during the course of macular degeneration. In early trials ACT's therapies appear safe so differentiating embryonic stem cells may indeed be a safe way to go to produce therapies that do not have clinically significant risk of teratoma formation [14]. Safety studies continue and whether the RPEs are effective to treat macular degeneration is as yet unknown.

Induced pluripotent stem (iPS) cells

Until 2006, the three main kinds of stem cells discussed above were the only ones seriously considered for clinical use at some future point. However, in that year a researcher in Japan named Dr. Shinya Yamanaka published an extraordinary paper [15] on a new type of pluripotent stem cell that he had produced from a rather ordinary type of cell called a fibroblast. He called the new pluripotent stem cells that had many of the same characteristics as embryonic stem cells by the name "induced pluripotent stem cells" or "iPS cells".

Yamanaka used a great deal of existing knowledge about embryonic stem cells and the ICM to come up with a panel of a few dozen candidate factors that he hypothesized might be "inducers" of pluripotency. By

"inducers" he meant factors that could change or induce ordinary cells such as fibroblasts, which are not even stem cells, into pluripotent stem cells through a process called "reprogramming". It was an audacious idea, but he was right.

By trying out different combinations or "cocktails" of these possible inducing factors he found that four specific ones together — Sox2, Oct4, c-Myc, and Klf4 — performed cellular alchemy when introduced into fibroblasts by turning them into iPS cells that were almost entirely indistinguishable from embryonic stem cells.

This inducing cocktail, which we can call SOMK (Sox2, Oct4, c-Myc, and Klf4) as an acronym, was forced into fibroblasts by infecting (also called "transducing" in the stem cell field) the cells with four retroviruses each encoding one of the four factors. The viruses, when all four infected the same fibroblasts, forced the cells to express the RNAs of Sox2, Oct4, c-Myc, and Klf4. In turn the cells have no choice but to then express the proteins for these factors, which are all transcription factors. Transcription factors are proteins that bind DNA at genes and turn genes on or off. In this case the introduced transcription factors together code for an embryonic stem cell identity and behavior by flipping just the right combinations of genetic switches.

Expression of SOMK changed fibroblasts into cells that were almost identical to embryonic stem cells (Figure 2.5). There was great excitement about the report of mouse iPS cells by Yamanaka in 2006 given the similarity of iPS cells to embryonic stem cells and the fact that their derivation did not require human blastocyst embryos, which are needed to make embryonic stem cell cultures as described above.

By the time Yamanaka reported human iPS cells the next year in a paper [16], several other labs also reported that they could make human iPS cells as well, surprising Yamanaka and the stem cell field with the speed of their competition.

Today most labs use the same SOMK cocktail (sometimes with slight variations) as Yamanaka to make iPS cells. Another lab, that of James Thomson of University of Wisconsin (who you will recall was the first to grow human embryonic stem cells) reported making human iPS cells with a bit of a different inducing martini: Sox2, Oct4, Lin28 and Nanog [17].

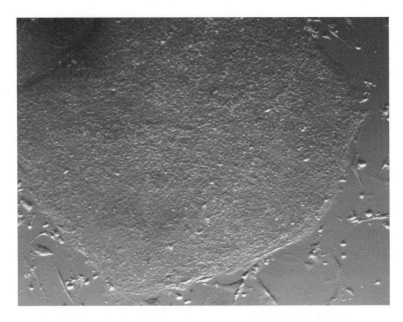

Figure 2.5. A human iPS cell colony growing on top of feeder cells. Notice the similarity to the human embryonic stem cell colony shown in Figure 2.3. Image Credit, Knoepfler Lab, Dr. Bonnie Barrilleaux.

The news of the production of human iPS cells even entered mainstream pop culture. Dr. Oz famously told Oprah and Michael J. Fox, a proponent of embryonic stem cell research, that the stem cell debate over the use of embryonic stem cells was "dead" on the Oprah show.[vii] As it turns out, Oz was perhaps overly exuberant about iPS cells as now a half dozen years later, it still remains unclear if iPS cells can truly replace embryonic stem cells. As a result the stem cell debate continues.

Since 2007, a whole host of methods have been reported to make iPS cells ranging from a panoply of different viruses as vectors to make cells express the reprogramming factors, to purified RNAs, to recombinant proteins. Small molecule chemicals akin to the drugs that many patients take in pills each day in some cases can replace one or more of the inducing or "reprogramming" factors as well.

[vii]http://www.bioethicsinternational.org/blog/2009/04/08/dr-oz-tells-oprah-fox-that-stem-cell-debate-is-dead/

How do these factors make ordinary fibroblasts turn into extraordinary iPS cells? Surprisingly, the details are still being worked out, but we have a good sense in general of what happens. Fibroblasts are one of the most common cell types in the body fulfilling mainly structural roles. In some limited cases fibroblasts can differentiate into other cell types such as fat cells or muscle, but generally fibroblasts are not considered stem cells and they express many differentiation-associated genes.

Fibroblasts also normally express c-Myc, but at low levels and these cells do not typically express the other reprogramming factors, which are mostly uniquely expressed in the early embryo in the ICM. When these transcription factors are forcibly overexpressed in fibroblasts, one major thing they do is to shut down differentiation-associated gene expression. What does that mean? In essence, SOMK at a molecular level tell the fibroblast, via turning just the right combination of specific genes off, that it is no longer a differentiated cell but instead is a pluripotent stem cell. Differentiation genes turn off, while pluripotent stem cell genes turn on, and the cell changes its appearance and behavior accordingly. At some point the fibroblast, which might have been isolated from skin, becomes nearly indistinguishable from an embryonic stem cell and in theory can differentiate with the proper stimulus into any mature type of cell in the human body.

A little iPS cell pre-history

We need to go further back in the history of cell biology and attribute credit where it is due that established the groundwork for iPS cells. There was a scientist named Dr. Harold (Hal) Weintraub at the Fred Hutchinson Cancer Research Center (or as many of us call it affectionately for short "The Hutch") in Seattle, where I did my postdoctoral studies. You can read more about him here on the Hutch website.[viii]

Hal was definitely one of a kind, visionary scientist. When I arrived at the Hutch in Bob Eisenman's lab to start my postdoc in 1998, people

---

[viii] http://www.fhcrc.org/en/labs/basic-sciences/weintraub-award/weintraub-bio.html

were still grieving Hal's death from a brain tumor 3 years earlier (see his NY Times obituary[ix]).

Hal was a revolutionary researcher in the area of genes and cell fate. Yamanaka won the Nobel Prize in 2012 for his work on iPS cells along with Dr. John Gurdon who cloned the first vertebrate (a frog).[x] While the Nobel Committee can award one Nobel Prize to three scientists at a time, in this case they only gave it to Gurdon and Yamanaka, leaving one space open. I firmly believe that if Hal were still alive he would have been the third person for that 2012 Nobel Award.

Why does Hal deserve some credit for the discovery of iPS cells?

Hal did pioneering studies of how genes influence cell fate. His models of how genes control cellular identity were exemplified by his lab's seminal work on MyoD, a powerful transcription factor that can direct cell fate toward the muscle lineage. Hal's lab's first paper reporting the existence of what would later be called "MYOD" for "MYOblast Determination gene" was truly revolutionary [18]. His team reported that introduction of a single defined factor, MYOD, induced fibroblasts to change into myoblasts (muscle progenitor cells) that could then differentiate into myotubes, which are muscle fibers that are the fundamental unit of functional muscle.

MYOD reprogrammed even non-fibroblastic lineage cells into the muscle lineage. This factor-induced change of cell fate should sound familiar to you as being similar to iPS cell formation, which would be reported first only about two decades later. What this means is that, in the 1980s Hal demonstrated a defined factor could induce direct reprogramming of cell fate. The Weintraub lab papers from 1987 and 1988 more fully fleshed out the MyoD story [19, 20]. In a perspectives piece published recently [21], Yamanaka himself also attributes some of the credit in the pre-history of iPS cells to Hal Weintraub.

Fast forward to 2013 and clinical trial investigation of iPS cell-based therapies in humans may start as early as late 2013 or 2014 by a Japanese group proposing to use iPS cell-produced RPEs to treat macular

---

[ix]http://www.nytimes.com/1995/03/31/obituaries/harold-weintraub-49-biologist-who-studied-cell-development.html

[x]http://www.nytimes.com/2012/10/09/health/research/cloning-and-stem-cell-discoveries-earn-nobel-prize-in-medicine.html?pagewanted=all&_r=0

degeneration,[xi] similar to ACT's work with embryonic stem cell-based RPEs discussed earlier in this chapter.

What are the possible advantages and disadvantages of iPS cells for future clinical use?

Relative advantages of iPS cells: Autologous use and no need for embryos

Because iPS cells can in theory be made from any patient's skin, the hope is that iPS cell-based treatments would be autologous and cells would be viewed by the body as "self" and not be rejected. This would be a big advantage of iPS cells over embryonic stem cells. This issue of immunogenicity or the extent to which the body's immune system reacts to stem cell treatments is discussed in more depth later in the book.

A second advantage of iPS cells is that while they look and behave so remarkably similar to embryonic stem cells (Figure 2.5), no embryo is needed to make iPS cells. As a result, iPS cells are considered to be a stem cell that has less ethical baggage than embryonic stem cells. However, this may be changing in a surprising way as fundamentalists are realizing that iPS cell technology hypothetically could be used to clone human beings in the future (more on this in Chapter 12).

Relative disadvantages of iPS cells: Teratoma, mutations, timing and cost

It is also notable that from a clinical perspective that much the same as embryonic stem cells, iPS cells also have the strong potential to form teratoma tumors. In fact, the teratoma assay in research labs is considered a gold standard assay for measuring and validating the pluripotency of putative new iPS cell lines.

Much the same as for embryonic stem cells, potential teratoma formation in patients is also a potential roadblock to the future clinical use of iPS cells and researchers are taking much the same approach as with embryonic stem cells of differentiating the iPS cells so fully that

---

[xi]http://blogs.nature.com/news/2013/02/embryo-like-stem-cells-enter-first-human-trial.html

ideally essentially none remain as undifferentiated iPS cells that can cause teratoma. Future pre-clinical animal and early clinical human studies will bear out whether this approach makes iPS cell-based therapies safe in humans. I hope this is the reality, but I worry that the field may be moving too fast.

Another concern with iPS cells is their propensity to acquire mutations during the reprogramming process, but to date it is unknown whether such mutations, which occur at a low frequency, have any real consequences for how the cells behave [22]. Nonetheless it is an important consideration that I believe may have been too rapidly dismissed by some in the stem cell field, while others contend that under the right conditions some iPS cell lines have no mutations.

iPS cells also have more immediately potential practical disadvantages: (1) they take a long time to produce and validate (approximately 6 months); and (2) they are relatively expensive to make. Estimates of cost range as high as tens of thousand dollars per clinical grade human iPS cell line. These two obstacles may make it more difficult for the truly patient-specific autologous potential of iPS cells to realized in large numbers of patients. However some, including Yamanaka, have proposed making large banks of iPS cells that could be given in an allogeneic manner.[xii] iPS cells from such banks would be "matched" to potential transplant recipients in the same kind of fashion that bone marrow transplants are matched.

Importantly, candidate iPS cells that researchers make in the lab are only rarely the "real deal". They are validated as such in a number of ways including the shape of the colonies they form (real iPS cell colonies have very distinct borders and are round or oval), their gene expression, their function (e.g. ability to form teratoma), and the presence of specific marker proteins (e.g. cell membrane proteins) on their surface. Validation of a human iPS cell line produced in my lab is shown in Figure 2.6 by staining living cells with a human embryonic stem cell marker called TRA-1-60. In the middle is one full round colony of perhaps a thousand cells and two portions of separate colonies can be seen at left with the rest of those colonies being out of the frame of the camera.

[xii]http://www.nature.com/news/stem-cell-pioneer-banks-on-future-therapies-1.11129

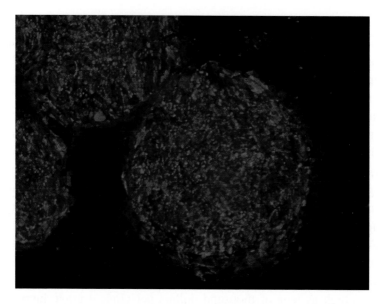

Figure 2.6. Candidate human iPS cell colonies are validated in a number of ways as real iPS cells including by living cell staining (red) for the human embryonic stem cell marker, TRA-1-60. Image credit: Knoepfler Lab, Dr. Bonnie Barrilleaux.

If the iPS cell production process only rarely makes real iPS cell colonies, what are the other cells produced as a by-product? Unfortunately, many of the other colonies of cells that are not iPS cells are likely cancer colonies, highlighting the similarity of cancer formation to the iPS cell reprogramming process. In fact, research in my own lab has shown that even real iPS cells have some striking similarities to cancer cells, raising serious clinical implications related to safety [23]. It was extremely difficult to get our paper on this work published and I believe part of the reason was that certain reviewers simply did not like the idea that iPS cells were similar to cancer cells. It is a shame that the reality that iPS cells have some similarity to cancer cells has largely been ignored by certain scientists in the iPS cell field.

An iPS offshoot: Direct Reprogramming or Transdifferentiation

Yamanaka's pioneering work on iPS cells got scientists thinking in more creative ways about cells. Stem cell researchers began to think that cells in general may be more flexible (what we in the stem cell field call "plastic") than ever imagined in terms of the various cellular identities that they can take on over time.

This innovative thinking led some to consider whether iPS cells were even necessary at all; perhaps we could change one cell type directly into another without the so-called "middle man" of iPS cells. For example, could one change the ordinary skin fibroblast directly into a neural cell that would normally be more at home in the brain, but without the intermediate iPS cell step? Some scientists thought that was possible.

A researcher named Dr. Marius Wernig led a team exploring this idea, a process first termed "transdifferentiation", but now more commonly called "direct reprogramming". In 2010, Wernig's team reported they could indeed transdifferentiate fibroblasts directly into neural cells, an amazing accomplishment [24]. It turns out that other forms of transdifferentiation had been reported earlier including both natural (stimulated during salamander limb regeneration [25], see more on potential limb regeneration in humans in Chapter 13) and induced by scientists [26]. Figure 2.7 gives an overview of how transdifferentiation works compared to iPS cell production.

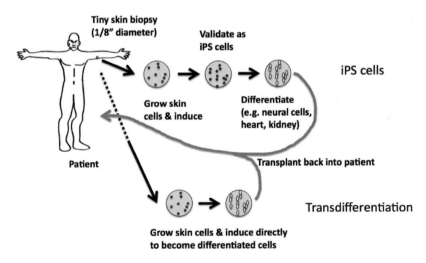

Figure 2.7. Model of how iPS cells are produced and could be used for autologous transplants in patients as well as how transdifferentiation-based approaches would be similar and different in some ways to iPS cells.

Other teams have more recently published studies on transdifferentiation induced in the lab. Just how promising transdifferentiation/direct reprogramming will become in the future for clinical use remains to be seen, but it is an sensational, cutting edge technology.

Summary

Ultimately, I believe that we need all the main kinds of stem cells and approaches discussed above. They each have unique advantages and disadvantages. If we are to help the maximum number of people who might benefit from stem cells we cannot throw one important type of stem cell out the window because of a minority opinion.

Knowing human nature, my impression is that many espousing the belief that embryonic stem cells are objectionable would change their mind if they or a loved one received a diagnosis of a disease that might only be helped by embryonic stem cells. Witness the conversion of Nancy Reagan to be an advocate of embryonic stem cell research after her husband's diagnosis with Alzheimer's Disease [27].

References

1. Kato, K, et al. (2012) Ethical and policy issues in the clinical translation of stem cells: report of a focus session at the ISSCR Tenth Annual Meeting. *Cell Stem Cell.* **11**:6:765-7.
2. Caplan, AI (1991) Mesenchymal stem cells. *Journal of orthopaedic research: official publication of the Orthopaedic Research Society.* **9**:5:641-50.
3. Roy, S, et al. (2013) Rare somatic cells from human breast tissue exhibit extensive lineage plasticity. *Proceedings of the National Academy of Sciences of the United States of America.* **110**:12:4598-603.
4. Schiavetta, A, et al. (2012) A phase II trial of autologous transplantation of bone marrow stem cells for critical limb ischemia: results of the Naples and Pietra Ligure Evaluation of Stem Cells study. *Stem Cells Translational Medicine.* **1**:7:572-8.
5. Karussis, D, et al. (2010) Safety and immunological effects of mesenchymal stem cell transplantation in patients with multiple sclerosis and amyotrophic lateral sclerosis. *Archives of neurology.* **67**:10:1187-94.

6. Ben-David, U, Y MaysharN Benvenisty (2011) Large-scale analysis reveals acquisition of lineage-specific chromosomal aberrations in human adult stem cells. *Cell Stem Cell*. **9**:2:97-102.

7. Prockop, DJ, et al. (2010) Defining the risks of mesenchymal stromal cell therapy. *Cytotherapy*. **12**:5:576-8.

8. Martin, GR (1981) Isolation of a pluripotent cell line from early mouse embryos cultured in medium conditioned by teratocarcinoma stem cells. *Proceedings of the National Academy of Sciences of the United States of America*. **78**:12:7634-8.

9. Evans, MJMH Kaufman (1981) Establishment in culture of pluripotential cells from mouse embryos. *Nature*. **292**:5819:154-6.

10. Thomson, JA, et al. (1998) Embryonic stem cell lines derived from human blastocysts. *Science*. **282**:5391:1145-7.

11. Noggle, S, et al. (2011) Human oocytes reprogram somatic cells to a pluripotent state. *Nature*. **478**:7367:70-5.

12. Baker, M (2013) Court lifts cloud over embryonic stem cells. *Nature*. **493**:7432: 282.

13. Moran, N (2011) European court bans embryonic stem cell patents. *Nature biotechnology*. **29**:12:1057-9.

14. Schwartz, SD, et al. (2012) Embryonic stem cell trials for macular degeneration: a preliminary report. *Lancet*. **379**:9817:713-20.

15. Takahashi, KS Yamanaka (2006) Induction of pluripotent stem cells from mouse embryonic and adult fibroblast cultures by defined factors. *Cell*. **126**:4:663-76.

16. Takahashi, K, et al. (2007) Induction of pluripotent stem cells from adult human fibroblasts by defined factors. *Cell*. **131**:5:861-72.

17. Yu, J, et al. (2007) Induced pluripotent stem cell lines derived from human somatic cells. *Science*. **318**:5858:1917-20.

18. Lassar, AB, BM PatersonH Weintraub (1986) Transfection of a DNA locus that mediates the conversion of 10T1/2 fibroblasts to myoblasts. *Cell*. **47**:5:649-56.

19. Tapscott, SJ, et al. (1988) MyoD1: a nuclear phosphoprotein requiring a Myc homology region to convert fibroblasts to myoblasts. *Science*. **242**:4877:405-11.

20. Davis, RL, H WeintraubAB Lassar (1987) Expression of a single transfected cDNA converts fibroblasts to myoblasts. *Cell*. **51**:6:987-1000.

21. Yamanaka, S (2012) Induced pluripotent stem cells: past, present, and future. *Cell Stem Cell*. **10**:6:678-84.

22. Barrilleaux, BPS Knoepfler (2011) Inducing iPSCs to escape the dish. *Cell Stem Cell*. **9**:2:103-11.

23. Riggs, JW, et al. (2013) Induced pluripotency and oncogenic transformation are related processes. *Stem cells and development*. **22**:1:37-50.

24. Vierbuchen, T, et al. (2010) Direct conversion of fibroblasts to functional neurons by defined factors. *Nature*. **463**:7284:1035-41.

25. Brockes, JPA Kumar (2002) Plasticity and reprogramming of differentiated cells in amphibian regeneration. *Nature reviews. Molecular cell biology.* **3**:8:566-74.
26. Zhou, QDA Melton (2008) Extreme makeover: converting one cell into another. *Cell Stem Cell.* **3**:4:382-8.
27. Check, E (2004) Bush pressured as Nancy Reagan pleads for stem-cell research. *Nature.* **429**:6988:116.

Chapter 3

Stem Cell Treatments: Applications and Obstacles

How exactly do we envision using all those powerful types of stem cells as medicines and what are the major obstacles in the way?

Just as there are many compelling, powerful ways to potentially use stem cells to treat patients, there are also numerous daunting obstacles in the way of making stem cell based-medicines a reality. In this chapter I tackle the main promising applications of stem cell technology for medicine as well as the key roadblocks that we face.

The Key Ways Stem Cells Can Be Used as Medicines

The most straightforward way that stem cells can be used as medicines is via what is called "cell therapy" in which stem cells or their differentiated progeny cells are transplanted to regenerate tissues, but four other areas are quite promising as well: immune modulation, secretion of so-called "trophic" factors, drug delivery, and organ replacement. The last of these is discussed in depth in Chapter 13.

All of these approaches are potentially very powerful, but their use in humans must be supported by data as evidenced-based medicine. What this means is that doctors cannot ethically conduct experimental stem cell procedures on people without first having compelling evidence that they are safe and effective as well as getting regulatory approval, for example from the FDA in the US.

Cell therapy

The cell therapy approach to stem cell-based medicine means that stem cells themselves or differentiated cells made from stem cells are transplanted into patients. The transplanted cells would repair or replace damaged tissues. Stem cell-based cell therapy is being investigated for an almost infinite number of medical applications. Because the normal job of stem cells is to grow healthy tissues, stem cells are "naturals" when it comes to cell therapy, although getting them to build the desired tissue type rather than a different one is a major consideration. For example, you would not want teeth growing in your hand instead of a new finger, right? Talk about a whole new way of thinking about the expression "biting the hand that feeds you."

Another issue for cell therapy is getting the cells to engraft and live in the right place. We also need the right number of cells. Too few cells may lead to a less than satisfactory outcome. Too many cells could destroy the tissue or organ in question.

Immunomodulation therapy

Stem cells can also be used indirectly to help patients via something called "immune modulation" or "immunomodulation". Stem cells not only build tissues, but also they secrete many soluble factors that influence the behavior of other cells. For example, if a researcher grows stem cells in a lab after a few days the media in which the stem cells were grown (called "conditioned media") becomes full of factors secreted by the stem cells even as the stem cells use up the synthetic growth factors that the researcher had added to the media when it was first made to support the growth of the stem cells.

Stem cells also secrete factors in vivo after transplantation. They release a continuous stream of factors to the cells and tissues around them. What this means is that in principle stem cells do not necessarily have to build new tissues to be helpful in treating pathological conditions. Stem cells may benefit patients with pathological conditions on some levels strictly via factor secretion. This mechanism is akin to the stem cells being doctors inside our bodies prescribing medicines to the cells around them.

The stem cell-produced factors could have any number of effects ranging from "waking up" sleeping endogenous stem cells to facilitating tissue repair to suppressing harmful immune responses and inflammation.

The latter mechanism whereby stem cells modulate the immune system has generated a great deal of excitement. Many human diseases even beyond autoimmune conditions have an inflammatory component. In the body's attempt to deal with disease or injury, typically there is a bystander effect whereby desirable, healthy cells are killed by "friendly fire" of the immune system.

During autoimmune reactions, which can be chronic in patients with diseases such as Multiple Sclerosis, the same kind of friendly fire events occur. If stem cell treatments can in essence turn down the activity of the immune system, the thought is that cells and tissues may get a break from the friendly fire of autoimmunity. Most often it is adult MSCs that are discussed as being used for immunomodulation therapy.

How would this work? Stem cells secrete specific factors (only some of which have been identified) that tend to tell immune cells to become less active. This approach has great promise, but critical questions remain about immunomodulation via stem cells.

If stem cells do indeed turn down the activity of the immune system, since almost all the stem cells given during transplants are rapidly eliminated by the body, **would patients require repeated stem cell treatments for the rest of their lives to keep chronic autoimmune conditions in check long term?** Such repeated treatments would be more likely to cause side effects and could collectively cost hundreds of thousands of dollars per patient.

In patients with already hyperactive immune systems is it not likely that stem cell transplants will be attacked and destroyed by the immune system even faster and more thoroughly than in healthy patients, greatly limiting or even completely negating therapeutic efficacy? The answer is yes and overcoming this obstacle will be key to the success of such treatments.

What are the risks associated with stem cell-based immuno-modulation? It is possible that immunosuppression by stem cells could make patients sicker due to a weakened immune response more generally leading to a higher rate of infections and possibly even cancer.

Overall, the use of stem cells to modulate the activity of the immune system is a very promising area of research with great clinical potential, but scientists and doctors still have much to learn.

Secretion of trophic factors

Stem cells not only secrete factors that modulate the activity of the immune system, but also they produce a host of other proteins and small molecules. Some of these secreted factors loosely fit into a class called "trophic factors".

Trophic factors are powerful biomolecules secreted by a variety of cell types that influence the behavior of other cells. Growth factors that stimulate cells to divide and grow fit into this class. Other trophic factors include angiogenic molecules that stimulate blood vessel growth and survival factors that block cell death.

In an injured or diseased tissue, stem cells (especially MSCs) secrete trophic factors that aid in repair and recovery. It is hoped that transplanted stem cells such as MSCs may do the same thing and in that way benefit the patient.

Via trophic factors, stem cells tell other cells to grow and to stay alive. Stem cells also signal for help by encouraging new blood vessels to grow into the damaged region to supply more nutrients and oxygen. The new blood vessels also act in essence as a pipeline for recruiting in endogenous cells that may aid in repair including potentially other endogenous stem cells circulating in the blood. Therefore, interestingly, one of the most promising ways in which transplants of exogenous stem cells may help patients is indirectly through stimulating endogenous stem cells to do positive things. At the same time there are risks as stimulating cell survival, proliferation, and angiogenesis may promote tumor formation as well. Therefore, trophic factors in theory have the potential to heal or harm depending on context.

Drug delivery

Stem cells seem to have a built-in homing mechanism that draws them to tissues that are damaged in the body. This homing mechanism is likely in place to assist endogenous stem cells in their natural job of helping to fix injuries. While in theory the stem cells themselves given as transplants may directly work to rebuild healthy tissues in part through this homing mechanism, clever scientists have come up with a second approach to take advantage of stem cells to heal: use stem cells as delivery mechanisms.

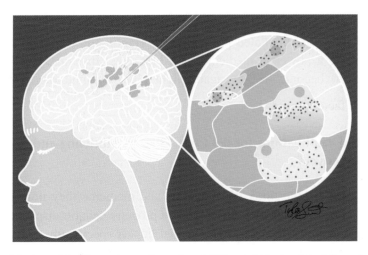

Figure 3.1. A model of how stem cells such as MSCs might be used to deliver drugs to specific sick cells (shown in brown) in the brain, making them healthy (light blue) again. The drug is shown as small blue dots. (Illustration by Taylor Seamount.)

In this way of thinking, since stem cells automatically go to injured tissues, they will be used clinically as drug delivery devices. Doctors will load the stem cells with medicines and send them off to treat specific tissues like micro-doctors or paramedics.

What could such stem cells deliver that would be medically helpful?

There are many possibilities. While stem cells naturally produce growth factors and immunomodulatory chemicals (discussed above) that could be beneficial, in addition stem cells can be designed to produce dramatically more of these molecules than normal. For example, for a given stem cell-produced natural growth factor, a designer stem cell might be readily manufactured that makes a thousand or a million times more of that factor than normal. In theory such a designer cell could be a powerhouse of healing.

Some diseases are caused by the body producing too much of a certain gene or protein or making a mutated protein that is toxic. In these cases designer stem cells may deliver inhibitory drugs to specific diseased cells in the body. The drugs would target and specifically block the activity of toxic molecules that are in excess or mutated (e.g. see the section on Huntington's Disease in Chapter 10) to lower their levels or activities. In the model shown in Figure 3.1, designer MSCs are injected into the brain of a patient with a neurological disorder such as Huntington's Disease, caused by a toxic mutated protein called Huntingtin. The MSCs carry and secrete a powerful medicine (tiny blue dots) that makes sick cells (in brown) become healthy again (light blue) by inhibiting the toxic Huntingtin.

Powerful Applications for iPS Cells: Disease Modeling and Drug Discovery

When most people think of stem cells and medicine they immediately imagine stem cells or their differentiated progeny being transplanted (i.e. cellular therapy). However, the potential impact specifically of iPS cells goes beyond their use in cellular therapy or the other applications mentioned above. While a medical future involving iPS cell-based cellular therapy was foremost on researchers' minds when iPS cells were first reported, more recently, a second powerful biomedical application has emerged for iPS cells: disease modeling.

In disease modeling, biomedical scientists use animals, tissues, or cells grown in culture in the lab to create a model of diseases separate from the human body. In this way, researchers can study the disease model to learn a great deal about why the disease occurs and what goes wrong.

They can also try out many different approaches for treatment in the laboratory without having to experiment on actual human patients. This is a critical distinction as working with human patients and experimenting on them is, rightly so, governed by strict regulations and often invokes complex ethical issues. Using disease models bypasses most of these roadblocks. It allows for discovery at a much faster rate than using actual human patients, although of course studies using human patients are still needed later on in the drug development process.

It turns out that modeling many human diseases has been difficult if not impossible for both doctors and scientists for more than a century. The differences between modeling and studying real human patients including the challenges of the latter can be illustrated by the example of Alzheimer's Disease, a devastating neurological disorder that afflicts millions of people. Scientists can and do study actual Alzheimer's patients of course, but such studies are complex, expensive, and limited in scope.

One such limitation is that scientists generally cannot readily study the cell biology of living brain cells from Alzheimer's patients because there is no practical and ethical way to isolate living cells such as neurons or pieces of brain tissues from actual Alzheimer's patients who are alive. Imaging techniques to study the living brain afflicted by Alzheimer's also have their limits. Once dead, the brains of Alzheimer's patients can still provide insight into the disease, but with major limitations such as cellular and tissue death that rapidly occurs after the patient dies.

In this sense scientists are operating somewhat in the dark when it comes to determining what goes so wrong leading to Alzheimer's and how to fix it. The same is true of dozens of other major human diseases. Living human patients are understandably reluctant to part with chunks of their brains or other organs. These limitations mean that for many diseases such as Alzheimer's scientists still do not understand what causes them, greatly limiting our ability to come up with new, effective therapies.

If one could model Alzheimer's Disease in a lab, a tremendous amount could be learned about its pathogenesis (a big word we use in science meaning how the pathology or disease condition arises). As it turns out iPS cells have the potential to create incredibly powerful disease models for Alzheimer's and almost any other human disease.

Continuing with the Alzheimer's example (but you can insert any disease here), using iPS cell technology scientists can and in fact already have created living neurons in the lab from Alzheimer's patients (reviewed in [1]). To achieve this amazing "disease in a dish" model, scientists typically take skin cells from a patient, turn them into iPS cells, and then differentiate the iPS cells into the desired type of cell that is most relevant to the disease in question such as neurons for Alzheimer's.

In this way, researchers have living models of human disease in a dish that can be used to study the disease in a fundamentally new, direct way never available before. For example, researchers can create pancreatic beta cells from diabetics via iPS cell technology and study the human beta cells in the lab. Beta cells are the cells that are lost or damaged during the progression of Diabetes that normally regulate blood sugar levels. In theory using iPS cell technology, researchers could make an entire mini-pancreas from a diabetic patient and study it in the lab. Of course in principle beta cells or a mini-pancreas could also be transplanted into diabetic patients to try to treat or cure them as well.

From iPS cells, scientists can make cardiac myocytes (the beating muscle cells of the heart) starting with skin cells from heart disease patients, neurons from Parkinson's patients, muscle cells from patients with muscular diseases, and so forth. All of this is possible with iPS cell technology, whereas up until the last few years scientists often had to wait until patients died and scramble to try to harvest living, but perhaps already dying cells from cadavers or work with limited tissues biopsies. iPS cells are revolutionary for increasing our knowledge about human disease via modeling.

In addition, this disease modeling application opens up another powerful door clinically. Scientists can "treat" the disease model cells or organs in the dish with panels of drugs to search for specific chemicals that revert the behavior of the cells back to normal. Such iPS cell-based drug screens are of great interest to big pharmaceutical companies and small biotech companies alike, which are all searching for new drugs.

In these ways iPS cells already look to have tremendous impact on medicine to help many people, without the iPS cells yet having been approved for clinical use in cellular therapies or introduced even into a single patient.

Stem Cells May Greatly Reduce the Need for Animal Research Via Modeling

iPS cells and other stem cells may also have applications in another way as well in biomedical research. I believe that animal research is crucial, but I am also an advocate of the notion that we should use as few animals as possible and only when necessary. Interestingly, stem cell research may be a key way in which to dramatically reduce the need for animals in research studies. Stem cells such as iPS cells not only can take the place of actual human beings in studies such as disease modeling, but also they can be used instead of actual animals such as rodents or larger animals.

A good example would be toxicity studies where in the future new drugs may be initially tested in stem cell-grown human organs in a dish in a lab instead of in animals. In fact, the human synthetic organ testing system may not only reduce the burden on animal models, but also be more accurate. For instance, imagine a drug, XYZ, which might have liver toxicity. In the future XYZ may be tested first by exposing human mini-livers grown from iPS or embryonic stem cell cells in the lab to different concentrations of XYZ in dishes. One drawback of potential stem cell-based modeling of this kind is that it does not take into account metabolism of drugs into new forms of chemicals that only occurs in living animals (e.g. via the liver or kidneys), but still this approach seems quite promising.

Lessons from Bone Marrow Transplants

Today the main stem cell treatment that is actually being used by doctors around the world and has been proven effective for decades now is bone marrow transplantation (also known today in various forms as "hematopoietic stem cell transplantation").

Interestingly, more than half a century has passed since the first demonstration in biomedical research labs in animals that marrow transplant was effective in growing a new immune system, but it took quite some time for scientists to definitively prove that bone marrow transplantation works to replace a person's entire immune system and blood cells specifically because of hematopoietic stem cells that reside in the bone marrow. In other words, bone marrow transplants are stem cell therapies, but scientists did not know that for sure at the beginning.

What exactly is bone marrow transplantation and why is it given to people? What can it teach us about other emerging stem cell therapies?

The history of this pioneering stem cell treatment traces back to research on cancers of the blood system — leukemias and lymphomas — as well as to research during the height of the cold war on trying to find treatments for humans exposed to potentially lethal radiation.

By definition at diagnosis, cancers that appear as solid tumors such as liver, breast, or prostate cancer of the kind that I myself had, can be considered either local or metastatic. Local cancers appear to the doctor to be limited to just one place and sometimes (but not always) are curable by surgery, which in certain cases is followed up by local radiation treatments and/or systemic chemotherapy ("chemo").

By contrast, metastatic cancers are far more ominous and patients diagnosed with metastatic cancer have a relatively poor prognosis. Because of the nature of the vascular system being ubiquitous throughout the body, leukemias and lymphomas are different from solid tumors in that they are by definition always metastatic from day one.

This intrinsic metastatic nature of blood cancers means that leukemias and lymphomas at diagnosis are spread throughout the whole body. As a result, these cancers cannot be treated effectively simply by surgery and localized radiation. In order to treat these cancers, most often patients must receive chemo infusions that are profoundly toxic to the whole body.

A devastating side effect of this kind of chemo is the rampant death of normal, vital stem cells. In order to have a good chance of killing all of the most aggressive cancer cells, the chemo must be so potent that the patient's non-cancerous immune system including the blood-forming hematopoietic stem cells as well as precursors to red blood cells and platelets are also totally destroyed. Fortunately, biomedical researchers found that the immune system could be restored by bone marrow transplantation. As a result, patients could have their leukemia or lymphoma eradicated and while their own non-cancerous immune system and blood stem cells would be destroyed along with the cancer, the bone marrow given to them post-chemo would often restore their immune systems.

Bone marrow is a unique tissue that lives inside the cavities in the middle of our bones. Unlike bone, the marrow is soft and contains a great diversity of cells including hematopoietic stem cells. It is a remarkably productive tissue, producing about one trillion new cells every couple days in humans. Note that this means that about one trillion blood and immune cells naturally die every day as well and need replacement. This highlights the key normal role of endogenous stem cells in tissue homeostasis in the body.

Researchers have determined that following a bone marrow transplant it is the stem cells in the marrow that can grow the patient a new immune system from scratch. Of course bone marrow transplants do not always work. In addition, there are many potential short and long-term side effects including secondary cancers and frankly, death. It remains a very high-risk procedure, but nonetheless, one that has saved many thousands of lives. The alternative for many patients is certain death.

For hematopoietic stem cell transplants, the stem cells are often isolated from the peripheral blood producing a treatment called more specifically, "peripheral blood stem cell transplantation" or PBSCT. Normally the number of stem cells floating free in the blood is low as they mostly reside in the bone marrow. For this reason, patients are given a growth factor called Granulocyte Colony Stimulating Factor (G-CSF) prior to harvesting stem cells from the blood as G-CSF greatly increases the number of stem cells circulating in the blood.

Today scientists, doctors, and patients are excited about using a diversity of stem cells for a much wider array of disorders beyond blood cancers and immune deficiency syndromes. For our purposes in this book, we can use hematopoietic stem cell/bone marrow transplantation as an example to which to compare other potential stem cell treatments.

Cautionary Lessons from Gene Therapy for the Stem Cell Field

As much as the stem cell field today can learn from the history and experience of bone marrow transplantation including its successes as a stem cell therapy, there are additional lessons to learn that are more sobering from other innovative, biotech fields. A helpful even if frightening, cautionary example comes from the gene therapy field.

In the early 1990s gene therapy seemed to be on the fast track to becoming a reality as a powerful, new type of medicine. However, gene therapy as a field was disastrously derailed, at least in part by moving too fast. This haste combined with a relative lack of knowledge due to the newness of gene therapy, led to several patient deaths including most famously that of Jesse Gelsinger.

After the deaths were proven to be caused by the gene therapy, there was a media firestorm. A story entitled "The Biotech Death of Jesse Gelsinger" by the *New York Times* was just one of scores of articles.[i] The

---

[i]http://www.nytimes.com/1999/11/28/magazine/the-biotech-death-of-jesse-gelsinger.html?pagewanted=all&src=pm

overwhelming reaction essential froze the field of gene therapy. Now two decades later it is no exaggeration to say that the gene therapy field is still recovering and in a "thaw" phase after an ice age of sorts.

What is gene therapy?

Many diseases are caused by mutations in specific genes. These mutations can be inherited or more rarely spontaneous. The idea behind gene therapy is to correct disease-associated mutations using genetic technology. In a prototypic gene therapy approach a corrective "transgene" (meaning engineered gene) is introduced into cells from a patient whose cells all contain a specific mutation. The transgene is designed to fix the mutation. The idea is that the cells with the corrected mutation will in turn restore normal biological function to the affected organ of the patient.

In one approach, the transgene is delivered to the patient's cells via transduction ex vivo (outside the body) with a virus such as adeno-associated virus (AAV) followed by returning the cells to the patient. Alternatively the transgene can be delivered in vivo inside the body directly into the target organ or systemically.

What went so wrong with gene therapy in the 1990s and what can the stem cell field learn from that experience to hopefully avoid similar problems?

In essence the gene therapies had unexpected side effects including cancer formation that killed patients. Based on their initial studies including pre-clinical data from animal studies, the teams conducting gene therapy at that time thought it would be safe, but it turns out that they were wrong.

There remain important, quite serious concerns about gene therapy even as it recovers as a field including its safety in patients, but also possible germline transmission of gene therapy transgenes to the children of patients. For the latter potential side effect, the concern is that the transgenes might find their way into sperms and eggs, and hence be inherited by the patient's children.

I saw a powerful talk in March of 2013 at the CIRM Grantee Meeting from gene therapy pioneer, Dr. Katherine High, who had cautionary lessons for those of us in the audience wanting to develop stem cell therapies.[ii]

[ii]http://www.ipscell.com/2013/03/blogging-the-cirm-grantee-meeting-wed-march-6/

One lesson for the stem cell field from gene therapy is that there will be unexpected effects of stem cell therapies. A high level of caution is in order. It is hubris or ignorance amongst proponents of extreme deregulation of stem cell oversight to claim that we know enough to define certain laboratory-grown stem cell therapies as definitively safe with our current, incomplete knowledge base.

Another message for the stem cell field is that studies in animal models often do not teach us what will really happen in human patients. We also need to essentially 'expect the unexpected' and take responsibility for what happens. We should soberly consider that the death of a single patient from a new biomedical technology is not only tragic for that person and their family, but can also potentially derail an entire field and delay future therapies. Such delays can in effect harm many more patients. In short paradoxically, by moving too fast the stem cell field may in effect slow the speed with which it can help patients through disastrous, but potentially avoidable negative outcomes. Proponents of deregulation of stem cell therapies want to weaken regulatory oversight to supposedly help patients more quickly, but in the end they may achieve the exact opposite result.

Why do stem cell therapies have the potential to harm? I find an analogy that is helpful to understand the risks of stem cell therapies is to "cellularize" (i.e. akin to anthropomorphize) pills. Imagine you swallow a pill and instead of disintegrating entirely into its molecular constituents in your stomach and intestines, it could divide, grow and become two pills. Then those two pills could become four pills, and so forth. Also consider that these hypothetic cell-like pills could migrate in your body in the bloodstream and perhaps even infiltrate your brain or other organs where they could grow. Anywhere the pills went they could also release some of the drug contained in them. In fact, they might even synthesize and release dozens of other drugs too. Neither you as the patient nor your doctor could control how the pill-cells acted once in your body. Perhaps this analogy gives you a sense of just how little control anybody has over stem cell transplants once they are given as medicines.

I worry that the stem cell field could soon find itself in a similar position as gene therapy in the 1990s if the proponents of stem cell deregulation prevail or because some people in the stem cell field have rushed to push their stem cell therapies into human patients before the time is right where we have enough information to justify the jump from pre-clinical to clinical studies.

Four Key Biological Roadblocks to Stem Cell Treatments

As with so many things in life, it is not so simple to just go out and get a stem cell procedure for whatever ails you. There are possible roadblocks to making safe and effective stem cell treatments a reality. There are also significant potential side effects and risks from stem cell treatments as alluded to in the previous section. Recognizing and understanding these challenges and roadblocks is of great importance for confronting them and overcoming the issues. Ignoring roadblocks is a recipe for disaster.

To become a true stem cell expert, you should know both the positives and the negatives. Ultimately, we need to consider all key elements of stem cells — good and bad — to realize the goal of mainstream, safe and effective stem cell treatments. I am optimistic that these issues will be resolved for stem cell treatments for many of today's most troubling diseases. Here I tackle the biological challenges to making safe and effective stem cell treatments a reality.

Immunity issues

When considering stem cell treatments, issues of immunity are critical. The human immune system has evolved to attack and destroy invaders in our bodies. Our immune systems are remarkably good at finding and killing anything foreign inside of us. The targets of our immune cells could be bacteria, viruses or parasites. In addition, because viruses infect cells and cause those cells to become essentially virus-producing factories, our immune cells are very efficient at finding and killing our own infected human cells as well. The immune cells will kill virus-infected human cells even though those are from the same body as the immune cells. If immune cells were not so good at this, we would all be dead from viral infections.

Conversely too much immune activity can also be deadly.

Our immune system normally leaves our own healthy cells alone so that we do not kill ourselves. One can see, though, that in human autoimmune disorders that sometimes our immune system attacks cells of our own bodies by mistake. Immune cells have somewhat of a hair trigger. If something about cells is not just right, immune cells will kill them even if immune cells otherwise realize that these are indeed its own cellular kindred from the same body. For example, virus-infected cells are recognized as trouble by the immune system and killed based on relatively subtle changes in the types of proteins on the infected cells' surface, a milieu that in some cases includes just a few foreign viral proteins amongst a sea of otherwise very normal, "self" protein.

Keeping these attributes in mind, one can see how transplanting stem cells into the human body could on many levels be troublesome from an immune system perspective. Any time one proposes transplanting stem cells from one person to a different person it is called an "allogeneic transplant". After an unmatched allogeneic transplant the recipient's immune system will attack the donor's stem cells as foreign and kill most or all of them (see more on what really happens during a stem cell transplant later in this chapter). This is why, for example, bone marrow transplant immune matching is so crucial.

How do cells recognize each other as either foreign or family (self)? Cells in essence have an identity code composed of multiple proteins that they express on their outer membranes, which is the part of the cell that is in contact with the outside world including other cells. This is to a great extent how cells talk to each other.

When cells touch each other, which interestingly happens all the time in the body naturally, they "read" each other's identity codes. It is sort of like having a secret handshake. If something is not quite right about a cell's code (by analogy that secret handshake or fist-bump is missing some key part like the jellyfish wiggle of the fingers at the end akin to tentacles), the immune system is called in to kill the cell.

Successful allogeneic stem cell transplants such as bone marrow or hematopoietic stem cell transplants between matched donors and recipients depend on and work because of the donor's cells having the same identity code as the recipient's cells. As a result, with a matched transplant the donor cells that are transplanted are recognized as "self" by the recipient's immune system and given a pass. In essence the immune system says, "You are one of us, you can live."

Other than bone marrow transplants, surprisingly most allogeneic stem cell transplants being conducted today by point-of-care clinics around the world are not between matched donors. As a result, for the vast majority of stem cell transplants of that kind today, most if not all of the transplanted stem cells are simply killed by the recipient patient's immune system in as little as one day, making such transplants illogical and futile. They are however quite profitable for the doctors and clinics performing the procedures at anywhere from ten to thirty thousand dollars per transplant.

Why then, besides pure greed or ignorance, do so many clinics and doctors still promote such unmatched allogeneic treatments to patients? They claim that stem cells are somehow sneakier than the average cell when it comes to immune recognition codes. This proposed so-called "immunoprivileged" state is argued to essentially mean that stem cells have an identity code that, while not the same as any given transplant recipient's cellular code, somehow achieves somewhat of a universal recognition as "okay". While stem cells and even differentiated cells made from stem cells have been proposed to be immunoprivileged in this way, this theory remains a controversial notion.

Importantly, even with transplants of one's own stem cells (called "autologous" as opposed to allogeneic from someone else), immune issues can still potentially arise. As a result, even if a patient receives a transplant of their own stem cells (e.g. liposuction isolated abdominal fat stem cells transplanted to breast or face for cosmetic reasons; see Chapter 11), the patient's body may still recognize those cells as foreign and kill them.

Why?

This autoimmune reaction can be due to a variety of reasons including contamination of the stem cells following extraction or during propagation of the stem cells in a lab. The stem cells can be contaminated with xenoproteins (meaning proteins from other species from the root "xeno" meaning foreign) via addition of supplements to the growth media (discussed more in Chapter 5).

One of the most common growth media additives for labs trying to expand stem cell numbers in a lab prior to transplant is, oddly enough, the serum of cow fetuses (fetal bovine serum; FBS). Despite the "ick" factor, for decades FBS has been used to stimulate cell growth in culture in the lab because (A) it is easily obtainable from farms and (B) it is enriched with growth factors. A growth factor is a protein or other small molecule that binds to the surface of cells and in many cases flips a switch telling that cell to grow. One of stem cells' favorite growth factors is called fibroblasts growth factor (FGF). It is worth noting that cells of almost all species of animals have the machinery in place to respond to FBS, which will trigger nearly any species of cell to grow. It is a powerful reagent and relatively cheap.

But there is a catch. How would you like to shake hands with a cow? The human immune system does not like it either.

Research has demonstrated that once human stem cells, for example, are grown in media containing FBS the cells are permanently contaminated with certain cow proteins that are antigens that stimulate attention from the immune system. As a result, human stem cells exposed to FBS are far more likely to trigger immune responses once transplanted.

As you can imagine during a cellular "handshake" to verify identity between two human cells, a bunch of cow proteins might make it akin to a hoof held out to shake a human hand. That experience will feel foreign and trigger an immune alert. Therefore, although the cow growth factors in FBS such as FGF fit like lock and key into receptors on human stem cell membranes, telling those cells to grow, other cow proteins stick to that cell's surface and tell the human immune system that that cell is foreign.

Alternatives to FBS have been proposed [2] including commercial so-called "xeno-free" media that still keeps human cells happy without the use of non-human products. Still many for-profit stem cell clinics grow their patients' cells in FBS anyway because it makes the cells grow faster and human serum, which in theory could be used instead, is both expensive and must be tested for pathogens such as HIV or hepatitis. Other additives to which stem cells are exposed to in a lab and that could be problematic include specific synthetic growth factors, which can also trigger immune responses. A potential immune-related problem for the clinical application of human embryonic stem cells is the use of mouse feeder cells, which contaminate the human cells with mouse antigens [3].

Another potentially disastrous form of contamination is when cells from two different people are accidentally mixed together. In theory stem cells removed from the body can be mixed up or cross-contaminated with another person's cells being processed in the same clinical lab or cross-contaminated during laboratory processing via things such as centrifuges leading to immune reactions after transplant.

The idea that autologous stem cell transplants are inherently safe and somehow never going to trigger immune responses is used as a selling point by non-compliant clinics. However, autologous does not necessarily equal safe (as discussed later in this chapter) and has proven to sometimes (albeit much more rarely) trigger catastrophic immune reactions. In one particularly troubling case a patient received both an autologous and an allogeneic treatment in Panama with a disastrous outcome due to an immune reaction [4]. In another case, a paper described how patients who received autologous stem cell transplants for limb ischemia (lack of blood and oxygen in a limb) had very severe side effects about half the time, leading to termination of the study because of safety concerns [5].

One reason why even autologous adult stem cell therapies may evoke immune responses is because if laboratories are not experienced and well equipped, significant fractions of the stem cells transplanted may end up being dead. You might think that dead cells would be ineffective yet harmless, but in fact they can cause problems. For example, significant amounts of dead or fragmented adult stem cells can release normally masked, intracellular antigens that evoke immune responses. This process is akin to how vaccinations work, triggering an immune response without the live virus present. Some proteins inside of cells are never intended to be exposed outside to other cells and are viewed as foreign for that reason.

Among stem cells, iPS cells were originally assumed to automatically overcome the immunity issues related to stem cell transplants since they could be used for autologous transplants. For example, in the scenario of an iPS cell-based transplant, a patient's own skin cells could be reprogrammed into iPS cells, differentiated into a specific cell type such as cardiac myocytes, and then transplanted back into the same patient. Such cells were assumed to then be recognized as "self" by the immune system.

The supposed inherent ability of iPS cells to be used to make "self" transplants for patients from whom they were derived is not entirely proven. In fact, one study initially gave some reason to doubt this key assumption [6]. They found in mouse studies that while mouse embryonic stem cell-derived teratomas were accepted as "self" by syngeneic (same, matched genetic background) recipients, teratomas derived from mouse iPS cells were rejected with a massive immune response.

Since the above study focused only on teratomas (tumor rather than normal tissues) it probably overestimated the likelihood of autologous iPS cells to elicit an immune response. Indeed, two additional newer studies have suggested that differentiated cells produced from iPS cells may not trigger major immune responses [7, 8] in syngeneic recipients. Each of these two newer studies have some limitations such as only being done in mice, but they are encouraging that iPS cells made from a given patient can likely be used to produce cells/tissues that can be given back to the same patient without being rejected by the immune system. Still, until real experiments are tried in actual human patients we cannot be sure and results are likely to vary substantially depending on the patient and which iPS cell lines are used.

Genome issues

The word "genome" means all the DNA in one particular cell or in all of the cells of one person. Your genome, for example, is your unique compliment of DNA, which is shared overall about 50% with your parents and siblings. If you have an identical twin, you share 100% of your genomes.

One genome-related concern about using stem cells or their derivative cells for stem cell therapies is the potential of the cells to accumulate mutations in their DNA. A mutated genome could change stem cell behavior and potentially the behavior of differentiated progeny or daughter cells of stem cells. Since scientists, doctors and certainly patients all want stem cells to behave in a predictable, consistent manner, DNA mutations are a bad thing all around.

We have all heard about mutations in pop culture such as in sci-fi or horror movies that have mutant monsters or aliens, but what exactly is a mutation? Our DNA or genome consists of a code of molecules called "bases" that come in four types: A, C, G, or T. Different combinations of hundreds or even thousands of these four "bases" (e.g. together constituting a gene) encode information that will tell cells how to behave. Mutations are abnormal changes in these codes that can in turn change how cells behave.

Probably because we are growing them in the artificial environment of the lab, stem cells expanded outside the body are under a great deal of stress and have a dramatically higher rate of mutations than endogenous cells in the body. The mutations can be as small as a single base change (e.g. A to C) or as large as deletions or duplications of millions of these bases at one time. Often they fall somewhere in between.

The gene is the fundamental unit of the genome and it is thought that mutations in genes are particularly fraught with potential danger. By analogy think if you are a messenger carrying a note to an army general. The note says "Fire!", meaning to attack the enemy, but for whatever reason the "F" gets changed to "H", and when you arrive, after reading the note the general tries to hire the enemy instead of shoot at them. A similar single base change in DNA, especially in genes, can lead to dramatic, unintended consequences in terms of cell behavior. By contrast, a smudge in the corner of the note in an otherwise blank region with no writing is unlikely to do harm. The same is true of DNA mutations that are away from genes.

Normally we have two copies of all genes. However, some cells under stress, such as cells being grown ex vivo in the lab, or cells undergoing the reprogramming process to turn a fibroblast into an iPS cell, can acquire larger mutations such as a gain or loss of copies of entire genes. As a result it is crucial to examine stem cells for these so-called "copy number variations" (CNVs). Some genes, called "tumor suppressors", protect us from cancer. If stem cells have CNVs in which they have lost one or both copies of a tumor suppressor, those cells are more likely to start acting similarly to a cancer cell. Conversely, some genes are called oncogenes and they tend to drive cancer formation if they are present at more than two copies. We need to know how many copies of these oncogenes are present in stem cells as well. CNVs with three or four or a hundred copies of oncogenes, which have been found in cells at times, could spell big trouble from a safety perspective for stem cell products transplanted into human patients.

An axiom of cell biology is that any stem cell that is grown in culture in a lab will inevitably accumulate mutations over time. The longer they are grown, the more mutations they will accumulate. Poor growth conditions by inexperienced lab techs can also increase mutation rates. For example, letting cells get too crowded (called "confluency") greatly increases the chance of mutations and immortalization.

Amongst all stem cells, pluripotent stem cells in particular have a relatively high propensity to acquire mutations while grown in the lab. For example, in iPS cells and embryonic stem cells, a whole range of mutations from small to enormous frequently occurs during culturing of cells in a lab [9-12]. Surprisingly, scientists at this point do not know the functional significance, if any, of most of these mutations and other genomic abnormalities. However, what we do know suggests that these alterations may confer a selective advantage during growth in culture to cells that are more cancer-like and those mutated cells can take over a group of cultured cells during the time that the cells are grown in the lab.

Importantly, adult stem cells also can contain and continue to acquire mutations in culture that may predispose them to behave in undesirable ways following transplant. Although the stability of the adult stem cell genome is intrinsically much higher than that of pluripotent stem cells, mutations are still an important consideration from a clinical perspective for adult stem cells.

Side note: Human genomic mosaicism

Stem cell studies, specifically experiments with iPS cells, have overturned the long-held dogma that each of an individual person's trillions of cells are all 100% identical at the genomic level.[iii] In fact, we all contain very small, but detectable populations of cells that significantly vary at the genomic level from each other. In other words, we are each mosaics. That mosaicism becomes evident during iPS cell production where subtle differences in the genomes of iPS cell lines all made from one person crop up.

Epigenome issues

The genome is not the whole story.

Another key element that influences stem cell behavior is called the "epigenome", which consists of a cell's epigenetic state.

The information stored in our DNA is not directly "understood", meaning functionally interpretable, by cells. In fact, cells are essentially blind, in a direct sense, to the information in DNA itself. Using a molecular equivalent of the "Rosetta Stone", all cells ranging from yeast to humans, must translate the information in DNA into a new language that the cell can use to read the instructions for what it is supposed to do.

The information in the DNA bases first gets translated into a related molecule called RNA, which is subsequently translated again but into a new kind of molecular language: that of proteins. Specific proteins are given names, often based on the name of the gene that they are made from or even simply made up by scientists themselves. Predominantly it is the proteins and also the RNAs that tell the cell directly how to behave. Going back to our analogy of the army messenger, imagine that his note must be translated not once but twice out of two different codes. The same kind of thing happens in cells going from DNA to RNA to protein.

[iii]http://www.ipscell.com/2012/11/surprising-human-genomic-mosaicism-means-not-all-your-cells-have-the-same-dna/

The process by which the cell makes RNA and protein from DNA is not surprisingly highly regulated and it is the epigenome that is the conductor of the process. Of the approximately 20,000 human genes in our DNA, only some of them are in the "on" mode actively making RNA and protein. Others are in the "off" mode. Still others are in between. The collective stream of information coming out of the translation of our DNA, as controlled by the epigenome, tells the cell what to do at any one given time: divide, differentiate from a stem cell to a neuron, crawl over there, commit suicide, and so forth.

One major part of our epigenome consists of a whole "sauce" of proteins (specific proteins called "histones") that glom onto our DNA like a strand of spaghetti. Without that sauce, our DNA would be like a long mostly straight strand of chromosomal spaghetti, but in reality DNA collectively is almost always covered with various proteins so it is wrapped up, curled and packed. Only small portions are opened or kept open to make RNA. These are in the "on" mode. The DNA binding proteins such as histones along with direct changes in the chemistry of the DNA itself through modifications called "methylation" are collectively what make up the epigenome.

The epigenome tells cellular machines to make RNA from the DNA or to not make RNA from the DNA or precisely how much RNA to make. It is the masters of the DNA so you can imagine the epigenome is very powerful and the epigenomic state of stem cells tells us a great deal about how they are going to behave. The study of the epigenome is called "epigenetics" or "epigenomics".

DNA is packaged with the whole host of epigenomic proteins with the primary type being the histones. Histone proteins are DNA binding proteins that form an octamer (group of 8 molecules) of two molecules each of 4 types of histones: H2a, H2b, H3, and H4.

When an octamer of histones is bound to DNA (the DNA is actually wrapped around the histone octamer like a strand of spaghetti looping around a meatball), the complex is called a "nucleosome", which is a fundamental epigenetic unit. How these histones are bound to DNA as well as their post-translational modifications (e.g. phosphorylation, methylation, acetylation, and so forth) constitutes yet another code. This code determines how the information in the DNA is translated into action to form RNAs and proteins as discussed above. The histone code is complimented by a second functional component of the epigenome mentioned earlier, DNA methylation, which tends to shift DNA into an inactive mode.

A key principle to understand is that while every cell in the body of one organism has the same genome (or nearly so excluding our small genomic mosaicism mentioned earlier), the cells all have very distinct epigenomes. For example, scientists often distinguish stem cells from non-stem cells by their epigenomes. While the genome of a stem cell and a non-stem cell from the same animal have identical DNA, stem cells typically have a signature epigenomic state. That epigenomic signature is not just handy for stem cell scientists trying to pick out stem cells, but also the reason it is there is because stem cells need different information streaming out of their DNA than the average cell. The epigenome of stem cells makes that a reality.

Cellular reprogramming to induce pluripotency and make iPS cells (discussed in the previous chapter) works by essentially re-writing the epigenetic code of the cells from a non-stem cell to that of a stem cell. Cellular reprogramming reworks the epigenomic code of a fibroblast to that of an embryonic stem cell so in essence what scientists are doing is telling that fibroblast "hey, look at your epigenomic code, you aren't a fibroblast, you're an embryonic stem cell so start behaving like one!" And remarkably, this actually works some of the time. All of the key iPS cell inducing factors — Oct4, Sox2, Klf4, c-Myc, Nanog, and Lin28 — work at the epigenomic level to influence gene transcription.

The epigenomic code is so powerful that it overrides other programming. The epigenome of a fibroblast, for example, is changed permanently to almost identically take on the features of that of an embryonic stem cell when a scientist makes iPS cells. The billions of bases of DNA that can be methylated or unmethylated along with the astronomical number of histone molecules (with their own compliments of modifications) and other proteins and RNAs bound to just one strand of the DNA, together comprise a system of almost infinite complexity. Therefore, changing this system from that of a fibroblast to that of an iPS cell with embryonic stem cell characteristics is a herculean task. Not surprisingly, sometimes epigenomic reprogramming is not perfect during iPS cell formation [13-16]. Researchers have reported a number of epigenetic differences between iPS cells and embryonic stem cells. The functional meaning of these differences is under intense investigation.

The adult stem cell epigenome is also dynamic and can vary in ways that influence the function of the cells. Adult stem cells, while sharing some epigenomic features with fetal, embryonic, and iPS cells, also have some unique elements. The epigenomic state of adult stem cells is certainly of great importance to how those cells behave (both in clinically desirable and undesirable ways), for example, after a transplant.

Notably, there is a panoply of epigenetic modifying drugs that have specific functions when used to treat cells. These actions can range from whole-scale changes in the entire epigenome of a cell to discrete changes in very specific elements of the epigenetic code. These drugs can powerfully enhance iPS cell formation, for example, and potently influence stem cell behavior. The use of epigenetic drugs to tailor stem cell behavior is an exciting, emerging area in the field and has great potential for clinical significance.

Overall it is crucial for stem cell researchers and physicians seeking to conduct stem cell transplants to keep the epigenome in mind and some have even proposed that the epigenome of every batch of stem cells intended for clinical use should be examined prior to transplant to look for potential harmful changes.

More broadly it should be noted that some leading stem cell scientists such as Yamanaka and Jeanne Loring are now inclined to believe that the three key issues discussed above (immunogenicity, the genome, and the epigenome) have already largely been resolved, but in 2013 most stem cell scientists remain concerned about these potential challenges.[iv]

Tumorigenicity

Stem cells are unique amongst the diversity of hundreds of human cell types. Almost every cell in the body is a non-stem cell and without some kind of laboratory intervention (e.g. making iPS cells from non-stem

---

[iv]http://www.ipscell.com/2013/05/jeanne-loring-on-reasons-for-optimism-on-clinical-translation-of-ips-cells/

cells), most of our cells will never be stem cells again although they all developmentally came from stem cells at some point.

However, there is one cell type that to our misfortune is uncomfortably similar to stem cells: cancer cells. In fact, the whole field of stem cells really started with studies of cancer (see more on that in the next chapter) and the specific subfield of pluripotent stem cells largely originated from studies of unique cancers called teratocarcinomas (relatives of teratoma, but malignant versions) that have cells with striking stem-like properties.

As it turns out, even "normal", endogenous stem cells are cousins of cancer cells. The different cellular parts such as DNA, RNA, proteins, cell membranes, and the epigenome of stem cells share some important similarities to those of cancer cells. It is unlikely to be coincidence that each of the key iPS cell inducing factors — Oct4, Sox2, Klf4, c-Myc — are either outright oncogenes or are highly expressed in cancers. In addition immortalizing cells (e.g. by inhibiting the function of tumor suppressor genes) promotes both cancer and cellular reprogramming.

If you think about it from a broad perspective, this similarity between cancer and stem cells, while disturbing from the clinical view of using stem cells for therapies, is not entirely surprising. The first job of stem cells is to grow our bodies and then later in adults it is to stimulate just enough growth of organs and tissues to either maintain homeostasis or repair injuries. Cancer cells really only know one job and that is to stimulate tissue growth too, just without the normal constraints in place. Stem cells promote controlled growth, while cancer cells drive uncontrolled growth.

From a clinical perspective, the familial nature of stem and cancer cells is arguably the greatest roadblock to making safe and effective stem cell therapies. It is not enough for a stem cell therapy to fix an injury (i.e. be efficacious); the stem cell therapy must also be safe.

Another indication of the strong similarity between tumor cells and stem cells is the fact that the most popular test of pluripotency for iPS and embryonic stem cells is teratoma formation, as mentioned earlier, which is inherently a tumorigenesis assay. In other words, paradoxically when scientists want to test the stem-like nature of their candidate pluripotent stem cells they most often analyze whether the cells can make a specific type of tumor (teratoma). Surprisingly, most types of stem cells such as iPS cells produced in the last few years have not been analyzed for their ability to cause malignant cancers (scientists often mistakenly just focus primarily on teratoma-forming ability of stem cells), so we do not know in many cases just how dangerous (or not) that a particular type of stem cell might be. A secret of sorts in the iPS cell field is that iPS cells can sometimes make malignant teratocarcinomas instead of teratomas during teratoma assays. iPS cells, embryonic stem cells, and adult stem cells have all also been shown in certain circumstances to cause other kinds of malignant tumors as well.

The importance of the cancer potential of stem cells is illustrated by the fact that biotechnology companies currently in Phase I or combined Phase I/II trials for embryonic stem cell-based therapies as well as those conducting pre-clinical studies leading up to future Phase I trials must have conducted such clinically-relevant safety studies (mostly, but not exclusively focused on tumor and cancer formation ability), as required by the FDA. Most new types of stem cells still have not cleared the hurdle of being shown to lack cancer-forming activity.

In addition to patients getting cancer as a possible side effect, potentially disastrous non-tumorigenic, but spurious tissue growth can also occur.

Cell Fusion and Confusion of Cell Identity

Stem cells have many unique properties and some are useful from a clinical perspective. However, certain attributes are more of a mixed bag having potentially positive and negative implications. One of these more complicated stem cell traits is something called "fusion", meaning that stem cells have a propensity to not just come up and hug or shake hands with other cells, but also fuse with them to become one new hybrid cell.

When a stem cell fuses with another cell the results are unpredictable. One possible outcome is that our new hybrid fused cell will simply die from the shock of the fusion. Imagine some person walked up to you and literally fused bodies with you to become a conjoined twin. A bit of shock, right? The same is true for cells that have undergone fusion. However, surprisingly, cells have an unexpectedly high tolerance for fusion.

Assuming our hypothetical stem cell/non-stem cell hybrid, fused cell survives the shock of fusion, what might happen next? One key question is whether the two nuclei of the now fused cell also fuse or not. If the nuclei fuse so that the one cell has one nucleus, the hybrid cell now has twice the normal DNA content, which can be a big problem if this cell subsequently tries to undergo cell division. Sometimes such cells can survive cell division and all of its daughter cells from then on may have double the normal DNA content, a condition called "tetraploidy". Other times the daughter cells inherit variable amounts of DNA from their hybrid mother cell, often leading to their death. If the nuclei of the fused cell do not also fuse, then that hybrid cell is now called "binucleated".

Whether the fused hybrid cell has one or two nuclei, its behavior is difficult to predict. It may act more akin to a stem cell if the stem cell programming dominates or alternatively it may behave more like the differentiated cell. Other times it takes on an entirely new personality such as that of a cancer cell. In short, fused cells are often confused, and the last thing one wants from a clinical perspective is a stem cell whose behavior cannot be predicted.

However, cell fusion may have its uses. For stem cell-based drug delivery there certainly would be no more direct way to get a drug into a target cell than to have the stem cell carrying the drug fuse with the diseased cell so that they then literally share their cellular contents. At this time the risks of cell fusion would seem to greatly outweigh possible benefits.

Why stem cells are so "fusogenic", meaning prone to fuse with other cells, and the mechanisms by which they fuse with specific cells and not others remains largely unknown. As knowledge is gained in this area, I predict that cell fusion may be something that can be inhibited or possibly controlled if researchers are trying to capitalize on fusion for a specific therapy.

In addition to the biological roadblocks discussed above, there are also aspects of human nature and more practical roadblocks that may slow progress in clinical application of stem cells. These kinds of roadblocks are discussed in the next section.

Bias

Another significant challenge to advancing clinical use of stem cells is research bias. Many human beings make remarkably good scientists and doctors, but even the best of them have biases, often unconscious ones. Patients also have a bias in that they understandably are looking for hope. A minority of patients ends up somewhat enamored of their physicians, even those taking tens of thousands of dollars from them. They see the doctors through rose-colored glasses as some kind of heroes. Patient bias (also called response bias) may be shaped by a desire to have a positive outcome or to please the doctor.

The nature of the group of patients that ends up receiving a stem cell treatment may also introduce bias, especially in a for-profit setting where only those who can afford an expensive treatment will get it. Stem cell treatments are in addition marketed to specific, select types of individuals, which can also introduce selection bias.

Investigator bias can be significant as well, particularly in the for-profit clinical setting where researchers may have a conflict of interest in getting positive results and generating income.

Building Rather Than Burning Stem Cell Bridges

The war-like attitude of some of the parties involved in the various debates over stem cell procedures also is not helpful for the process of making safe, ethical, and effective stem cell treatments a reality. The take-no-prisoners approach and use of propaganda by both proponents of stem cell deregulation and opponents of embryonic stem cell research, together tend to push constructive dialogue out the window. Instead, these people launch personal attacks on anyone who disagrees with them.

After two and a half years as a stem cell blogger, my impression in 2013 is that this kind of antagonism helps no one and hurts the stem cell field. Instead, I have adopted the exact opposite approach. I reach out to those with whom I disagree and try to build bridges with them. It does not always work. Admittedly, I have at times burned a bridge or two myself over my concern for patient safety, but overall I believe my efforts to build bridges among many diverse people in the stem cell field have had a positive impact.

Such bridge building has included hosting debates on my blog between people seemingly on opposite sides of issues. For example, Dr. Christopher Centeno of Regenerative Sciences Inc., who has backed stem cell regulatory changes, and Doug Sipp, an advocate of a relatively higher degree of stem cell regulatory oversight debated on my blog.[v] I have also hosted and participated in an ongoing dialogue with the Texas stem cell clinic, Celltex,[vi] a conversation that I have posted on my blog.

In addition, I did an interview with Dr. Ricardo Rodriguez, President of an industry-sponsored stem cell oversight group, the International Cellular Medicine Society (ICMS).[vii] I later posted my public recommendations on how ICMS could improve itself, indicating how crucial it is to tie bridge building with accountability.[viii] I also regularly communicate with leaders in the for-profit adult stem cell world even though we disagree on a number of issues. Communicating respectfully and working together is clearly the better way to help patients and make progress, while a war-like approach helps no one.

One of the most challenging types of roadblocks to stem cell therapies is paradoxically an area that gets relatively little attention: practical issues. By practical challenges to stem cell therapies I mean non-scientific reasons why we may have difficulty or even fail to get stem cell treatments to patients.

---

[v] http://www.ipscell.com/2012/05/interviews-with-centeno-and-sipp-on-key-case-on-fda-authority-over-stem-cells/
[vi] http://www.ipscell.com/2012/10/celltex-its-irb-provider-both-get-serious-fda-warning-letters-celltex-response-to-my-inquiry/
[vii] http://www.ipscell.com/2012/05/icms-president-rodriguez-interview-on-adult-stem-cell-regulatory-issues/
[viii] http://www.ipscell.com/2012/05/recommendations-to-icms-for-improved-practices/

Practical issues I: Cost

The primary practical roadblock to developing stem cell treatments is cost. Stem cell research is extremely expensive and its progress tracks with available funding. Costs come in two main forms: therapeutic and research. Both are discussed below.

Therapeutic cost

Stem cell therapies are very expensive. For example, unlicensed stem cell interventions already being offered by point-of-care, for-profit clinics charge on average about $20,000 each in 2013. The clinics also often recommend multiple interventions, but frequently do not mention this until the patient has already received one. Patients have spent above $100,000 for a course of stem cell interventions over a few years. Increasingly in the world of adult stem cell clinics, one intervention is now considered not enough. Some people receive dozens. Future, FDA-approved stem cell treatments are likely to be very expensive too, a point often mentioned by dubious, for-profit clinics advocates.

Side effects from non-compliant stem cell interventions could lead to enormously expensive acute medical care (think trips to the ER and hospitalization). Imagine if someone made the analogy that heart surgery would be cheaper if it did not have to be regulated. Would anyone accept such an argument? I do not think so. I believe the same expectations of oversight must apply to stem cell-based medical procedures.

The anticipated high costs of emerging stem cell therapies such as iPS cells (I predict these might cost around $100,000 per treatment for an autologous therapy) are important to consider from a public health perspective. One of the most troubling effects of the high potential costs of stem cell therapies is that they could become a medical innovation mostly available to relatively rich people.

Research and trial costs: Funding issues

In order to try to make as many of these potentially powerful stem cell treatments that we are discussing in this book a reality, an enormous amount of research is necessary. The stem cells and differentiated cells made from them must be studied at many levels ranging from basic science into how they work to pre-clinical studies to clinical studies. Collectively this research costs millions of dollars for just one type of stem cell product intended to treat one condition. It is not unusual for such costs to go into the tens or even hundreds of millions of dollars over time to translate a therapy to the point where patients receive it.

Where does the money come from to support this research?

Outside of the for-profit clinic and biotech industry that rely on investors, public agencies and private foundations provide the money for significant amounts of stem cell research. In the stem cell field, NIH supports a great deal of research. For example, my own lab has an NIH grant to study embryonic stem cells and iPS cells. State agencies such as CIRM,[ix] which funds some of my lab's research, also provide funding of stem cell research.

Stem cell research is very expensive and more funding is needed at the national level to push this compelling new medical technology forward to help patients. But as costly as stem cell research might seems, it is also essential to point out that chronic and acute diseases are dramatically more expensive than stem cell research, costing the US alone trillions of dollars a year.

Practical issues II: Timing

Much the same as for other kinds of medical procedures and medicines, the potential of stem cell treatments depends on them being available to patients when they need them. Acute injuries in particular are challenging to treat using stem cells, unless the stem cell therapies in question are prepared in advance in bulk and cryopreserved to be ready for almost immediate use.

By definition such therapies would most likely have to be allogeneic in nature. Alternatively, patients could in theory bank their own adult stem cells, iPS cells or specific differentiated cells produced from iPS cells (e.g. neural progenitors, heart muscle cell progenitors, etc.) in

---

[ix]http://www.cirm.ca.gov/

advance. However, such banking is likely to be quite expensive raising the issue of costs and accessibility.

A proposed alternative to making iPS cells from scratch individually for each patient who might need them is to make "universal" iPS cell banks that have a wide variety of iPS cells that would be genetically compatible (i.e. recognized as self) with most human beings. iPS cell banks of this kind could in theory be used as a basis to give patients allogeneic, but matched transplants much the same as matched bone marrow transplants.

The practicality of making such banks is unclear and just how much "coverage" of the human race would be achieved is questionable. People with unusual genetic backgrounds would be less likely to be covered by such banks, as their cellular identification codes discussed earlier in the immunity section are rare. As a result an important ethical question is whether such banks would in effect discriminate against minorities. Even to develop a clinical grade, validated iPS cell bank that "only" covers 90% of human beings would likely cost tens of billions of dollars.

What Really Happens to Transplanted Stem Cells: More Challenges

Post-transplant of stem cells, we have no control of them

What really happens to stem cells or differentiated cells made from stem cells that are transplanted into a patient? Once these cells, which have spent anywhere from hours to weeks (or even years if frozen) in a lab environment, are injected into a person, what do we know about what happens next?

As it turns out, we know almost nothing about what stem cells do immediately after a transplant, a remarkably important gap in the field. Part of the reason for this gap is that it is extraordinarily difficult to track transplanted stem cells in the body of a patient. A good analogy would be trying to track a million salmon that you released into the Pacific Ocean. Not an easy task and unlike salmon, stem cells do not return to any one given spot predictably.

It is clear that once cells are transplanted into a patient, nobody has any control over them at all. The cells are free to do whatever their molecular programming and the host body tells them to do. The only exception to this would be if scientists genetically modify the stem cells prior to transplant to include a so-called "suicide" gene into them [17]. Stem cells with a suicide gene can be killed by giving a patient a drug should a problem arise. However, the introduction of a suicide gene into a stem cell population, which amounts to a genetic modification (hence this would be both a stem cell and gene therapy stem cell product requiring more regulatory oversight), may introduce its own risks and it is not clear that all suicide gene-containing stem cells in a population of millions or billions of cells would in fact die on command.

Lessons from the dead: Transplanted adult stem cells generally fail to engraft

One way to learn more about what happens to transplanted stem cells is to study dead patients who had at some point in their lives received a stem cell transplant. Such autopsy studies are rare, but quite informative. A team led by Dr. Katarina LeBlanc published a key paper on autopsy data from patients who had received allogeneic MSC transplants [18]. They analyzed the organs of 18 corpses of stem cell transplant recipients at autopsy for the presence of the DNA of the transplanted MSCs (distinct from the recipients' DNA since these were non-matched transplants).

The researchers found very limited engraftment of MSCs in the dead patients' bodies. The level of engraftment also seemed lower in patients who had their stem cell transplants at a greater length time prior to their deaths suggesting a progressive removal of transplanted cells from their bodies over time.

Since the level of engraftment was so low and it did not correlate with the clinical outcome in the patients, these findings support the idea that transplanted adult stem cells function via a transient, so-called "hit and run" mechanism to potentially aid patients, assuming one believes that the allogeneic MSC transplants of today and the recent past do in fact have any benefit at all. Encouragingly from a safety perspective, none of the 18 bodies showed any evidence of MSC-based tumor formation. The authors conclude, "The lack of sustained engraftment limits the long-term risks of MSC therapy", but I would say that it also greatly limits the potential benefit of MSC therapy too.

Almost certain death awaits nearly 100% of transplanted cells

One helpful and fun analogy is that transplanted stem cells are like pets (domesticated cells used to living in a lab, an idea explored further in Chapter 5) released or who wander into the wild of the universe of trillions of cells of a human body.

How does your pet dog Rover fare if he runs away at Yellowstone National Park as opposed to living his normal daily life at home? Most of the time he will die in the wild of course. He might survive in rare cases, but most likely only if his wild instinct starts taking over. He learns to hunt and avoid predators such as wolves. He finds shelter.

After "domesticated" laboratory stem cells are transplanted into the wild of the human body, what happens first? I will take the hypothetical example of IV transplantation of 100 million stem cells to address this question. The first thing that happens is that the cellular trauma of being transplanted into the blood stream likely kills a significant fraction of the stem cells. Going from growing in media designed to make them happy in the relative stability of a lab into a patient's flowing blood stream (or any other specific tissue in vivo) is an enormous shock. It may be sort of like what happens when you run from a sauna and jump into an icy lake, except multiply the shock by 10-fold.

Blood and cell culture media are very different. The pH is different between the two, the temperature may be a degree or two different, the salt concentration outside the cell is quite different, and there is a difference in pressure. Further, there are certainly going to be some immune cells realizing that the transplanted cells are foreign even if a full immune response is not initiated because of transient immune suppression via drugs given to patients or because of an autologous setting or immunoprivilege. These immune cells are akin to the predatory wolves in our example of Rover the dog who is loose in Yellowstone. They are fierce hunters who may track down our pet.

Despite all of this, let us accept for the moment the premise that half of the transplanted stem cells (or their transplanted differentiated progeny) survive this initial shock so that there are 50 million living transplanted cells now flowing through the patient's blood stream within hours of the transplant. The number could be far lower, but we will work with this figure.

What happens next?

Research suggests that most of the stem cells get filtered out in the lungs, where they simply die or are actively killed by immune cells [19]. The likely explanation for this removal process is simply that stem cells, with the exception of rare hematopoietic or blood stem cells, are not supposed to be in blood and the body knows this so it kills them. The unusual, harsh environment of the lung may also passively kill large numbers of transplanted cells as well. Other transplanted stem cells may end up in the liver or kidney, where they suffer a similar fate. All of this death and killing likely happens in a matter of days or a few weeks, leaving perhaps as few as only thousands of living stem cells out of those original 100 million injected stem cells.

A minority of the remaining cells may have a chance to engraft into an organ or survive for a short period of time riding around in the blood stream. Their odds of survival are of course relatively higher in an autologous setting. Most stem cells from an unmatched allogeneic transplant that survive the first few days or weeks of death and destruction, will be hunted down by the recipient's immune system as Rover will be followed by the wolves.

What if stem cells are transplanted not in the blood stream by IV injection, but instead within a specific tissue or organ such as the spinal cord or the knee joint? The survival rate is thought to be relatively much higher in this scenario, but many questions remain. The data is sparse.

A key issue with local, tissue-based injection of stem cells is the degree to which the stem cells will migrate. Cell migration after transplant is a double-edged sword. In some sense you do not want the stem cells to stay exactly where you put them. You want them to migrate locally specifically to the region of injury and do their work as little micro-doctors to heal. On the other hand you do not want the cells to go too far (e.g. to exit the target tissue entirely) because they could end up doing the wrong thing if they are in the wrong place. For example, you do not want fat stem cells in the brain.

More broadly, regardless of the mode of transplant of stem cells, the bottom line is that once cells are transplanted, they will do whatever their molecular instructions and the surrounding environment tells them to do, assuming they can survive. They will go where they please and where the body allows. And at this point, the field is so new we do not know much about how this will all play out.

Stem Cell Capsule

An intriguing, more controlled approach to stem cell-based therapies that may prove safer and more predictable is using a novel method called encapsulation. In this application, stem cells or their differentiated progeny are not injected into the body simply floating around individually in liquid, but rather are first placed inside of an engineered capsule. The capsule is permeable to molecules such as oxygen and proteins, but impermeable to cells. Unlike an encapsulated drug that is designed intentionally so the capsule dissolves to release the drug over a given time period, a stem cell capsule is designed to be rugged and stable, keeping the stem cells in and other cells out.

A company called Viacyte is developing an allogeneic, embryonic stem cell-based therapy for Diabetes that is encapsulated in this way. Embryonic stem cells are first differentiated in the lab to produce insulin-secreting human beta cells, which are then embedded in the capsule. The capsule would then be implanted in the body of a Diabetes patient.

Human studies of this therapy have not yet occurred, not even in clinical trials, but they are planned in as little as a few years. In mice, however, pre-clinical studies suggest that the encapsulated cells sense blood sugar levels and can maintain a relatively balanced level of glucose in the blood.[x] In essence, this cutting edge technological innovation is akin to a mini-pancreas.

---

[x]http://viacyte.com/products/vc-01-diabetes-therapy/

In the case of the Viacyte encapsulated therapy, there is control over the allogeneic transplanted cells since they, in theory at least, cannot escape the capsule (and even if they did the immune system of the host would likely kill them). In addition, if trouble arises, the capsule could even be removed by doctors if need be. As a result encapsulated therapies may be reversible unlike the standard stem cell therapies of today in which stem cells suspended in media are injected into tissues or bloodstream to move about the body willy nilly. The capsule could also be replaced every few years with a "fresh" one as needed.

As the field of regenerative medicine advances, we will learn a great deal more about how transplanted cells behave in patients. In the mean time we wait to see what the earliest ongoing studies teach us.

Summary

The predominant ways to use stem cells as therapies that I discussed earlier are creative approaches to medicine. I expect that even more applications will be developed in the future that will continue to astound and provide us all with greater hope. Stem cells have enormous potential to make our lives better, but we also face major obstacles. As the stem cell field moves forward and becomes ever more embedded in popular culture, we would be wise to balance our expectations and temper our exuberance with the realities of the stem cell world. Still, it seems reasonable to me to be very excited. I know I am.

References

1. Choi, SHRE Tanzi (2012) iPSCs to the rescue in Alzheimer's research. *Cell Stem Cell*. **10**:3:235-6.
2. Naaijkens, BA, et al. (2012) Human platelet lysate as a fetal bovine serum substitute improves human adipose-derived stromal cell culture for future cardiac repair applications. *Cell and tissue research*. **348**:1:119-30.
3. Halme, DGDA Kessler (2006) FDA regulation of stem-cell-based therapies. *N Engl J Med*. **355**:16:1730-5.
4. Alderazi, YJ, SW CoonsK Chapman (2012) Catastrophic demyelinating encephalomyelitis after intrathecal and intravenous stem cell transplantation in a patient with multiple sclerosis. *Journal of child neurology*. **27**:5:632-5.

5. Jonsson, TB, et al. (2012) Adverse events during treatment of critical limb ischemia with autologous peripheral blood mononuclear cell implant. *International angiology: a journal of the International Union of Angiology.* **31**:1:77-84.

6. Zhao, T, et al. (2011) Immunogenicity of induced pluripotent stem cells. *Nature.* **474**:7350:212-215.

7. Araki, R, et al. (2013) Negligible immunogenicity of terminally differentiated cells derived from induced pluripotent or embryonic stem cells. *Nature.*

8. Guha, P, et al. (2013) Lack of Immune Response to Differentiated Cells Derived from Syngeneic Induced Pluripotent Stem Cells. *Cell Stem Cell.*

9. Mayshar, Y, et al. (2010) Identification and classification of chromosomal aberrations in human induced pluripotent stem cells. *Cell Stem Cell.* **7**:521-31.

10. Hussein, SM, et al. (2011) Copy number variation and selection during reprogramming to pluripotency. *Nature.* **471**:58-62.

11. Laurent, LC, et al. (2011) Dynamic changes in the copy number of pluripotency and cell proliferation genes in human ESCs and iPSCs during reprogramming and time in culture. *Cell Stem Cell.* **8**:106-18.

12. Gore, A, et al. (2011) Somatic coding mutations in human induced pluripotent stem cells. *Nature.* **471**:63-67.

13. Lister, R, et al. (2011) Hotspots of aberrant epigenomic reprogramming in human induced pluripotent stem cells. *Nature.* **470**:68-73.

14. Pick, M, et al. (2009) Clone- and gene-specific aberrations of parental imprinting in human induced pluripotent stem cells. *Stem Cells.* **27**:2686-90.

15. Polo, JM, et al. (2010) Cell type of origin influences the molecular and functional properties of mouse induced pluripotent stem cells. *Nat. Biotechnol.* **28**:848-855.

16. Stadtfeld, M, et al. (2010) Aberrant silencing of imprinted genes on chromosome 12qF1 in mouse induced pluripotent stem cells. *Nature.* **465**:7295:175-81.

17. Schuldiner, M, J Itskovitz-EldorN Benvenisty (2003) Selective ablation of human embryonic stem cells expressing a "suicide" gene. *Stem Cells.* **21**:3:257-65.

18. von Bahr, L, et al. (2012) Analysis of tissues following mesenchymal stromal cell therapy in humans indicates limited long-term engraftment and no ectopic tissue formation. *Stem Cells.* **30**:7:1575-8.

19. Schrepfer, S, et al. (2007) Stem cell transplantation: the lung barrier. *Transplantation proceedings.* **39**:2:573-6.

Chapter 4

Stem Cell Models: Past, Present, and Future

The Discovery of Stem Cells

There is an intriguing history to stem cell research.

There was no one single discoverer of stem cells. In fact there were quite a few true pioneers who helped launch the field starting as early as the 1800s. The "discovery" of stem cells was an ongoing team effort over a period of more than a century and there is plenty of credit to go around. Some of this history is covered in an article in my favorite stem cell journal, *Cell Stem Cell* [1], but there is a good deal more to the story as well.

In 1908, a Russian histologist, Alexander Maksimov (Maximow), used the phrase "stem cell" as part of his model of hematopoiesis. This is often incorrectly cited as the first mention of stem cells. Even earlier than 1908 other scientists conceived of the notion of single so-called primitive cells (meaning stem cells) producing tumors or organs.

In 1905, Dr. Artur Pappenheim drew a very powerful model of stem cell function and differentiation (Figure 4.1). This model seems amazingly prescient and accurate to this day more than a century later. In the very middle is the multipotent stem cell. We will go through this model more a bit later on in the chapter.

Going further back, Dr. August Weismann discussed stem cells using the term "germ plasm" in 1885. As early as 1868, German scientist Ernst Haeckel published models of stem cell function and referred to the cell in German as "Stammzelle", which means "stem cell" [1].

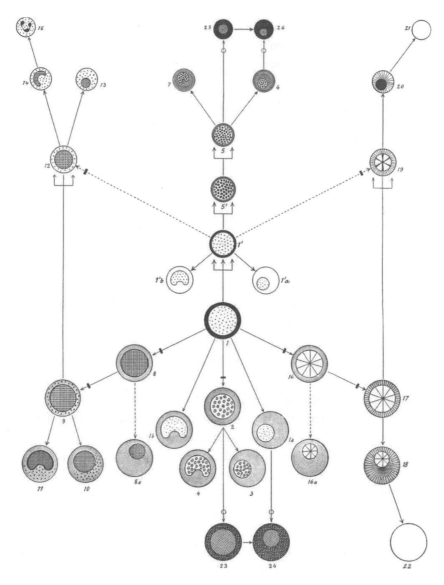

Figure 4.1. The Pappenheim model of hematopoietic stem cell function and differentiation. The small cell in the middle (with the trident like arrow coming up out of it) is the key stem cell [2]. Other differentiated and progenitor cells that are produced from the stem cell are shown as additional circles with different shading patterns and other distinguishing features. Indirectly or directly the stem cell gives rise to all the other cells shown.

What this means is that 100 to almost 150 years ago scientists presented evidence that stem cells existed, were germinal in nature, and were undifferentiated. In many cases, they even called them "stem cells" even if not in English.

What about more recent stem cell history?

There is an online public database of biomedical research articles called Pubmed[i] that is a very helpful tool for learning about stem cells. I highly recommend it to you. A simple Pubmed search shows that the first research paper in this database with the phrase "stem cell" in English in the title was by a scientist name MS Arrick in 1946, entitled "Stem cell lymphoma of the newborn" [3].

However, while science papers may be focused on a certain topic such as "stem cells", paradoxically they often may not mention that topic by name in the title so we have to dig a little deeper. Another Pubmed search shows that the first paper with the phrase "stem cell" in the abstract (the short summary that begins science research articles) was published much earlier in 1932. Dr. Florence Sabin was the first author of this very early stem cell paper [4]. For more on this incredible, pioneering woman scientist, see my tribute to her.[ii]

The abstract of Sabin's paper clearly indicates that their data support the notion that hematopoietic stem cells exist and are damaged by radiation. Sabin writes in the first part of the abstract (emphasis mine):

> "The observations in this work suggest that with certain doses of radioactive material, the fundamental damage in the lymphoid tissues is to the stem cell and that the damage is to the chromatin of the nuclei of these cells. The erythroid tissues are apparently less susceptible to radioactive material than the lymphoid tissues but an original anemia of secondary type from peripheral destruction may eventually be changed to one of primary type through decreased maturation of primitive cells in

---

[i] http://www.ncbi.nlm.nih.gov/pubmed/advanced
[ii] http://www.ipscell.com/2012/04/dr-florence-sabin-great-american-scientist-and-trailblazer-for-women-in-science/

the marrow. The damage of lymph nodes and bone
marrow leads to atrophy of these organs...."

In normal non-scientific English, what does this mean?

Sabin and colleagues (1) identified normal blood stem cells,
(2) indicated that radiation damages the DNA of the stem cells, and
(3) concluded that impaired differentiation of the stem cells contributes
to anemia. Therefore, this 1932 paper says that there are undifferentiated
hematopoietic stem cells in the marrow and they are functional.

Note that this entire 1932 paper is available to the public as a PDF if
you would like to read it.[iii] I find it interesting how an 80-year old paper
has much in common with today's science papers in terms of style and
sophistication, but also has some unique attributes. Note that Sabin
writes about stem cells in an authoritative way in this paper.

A later 1936 article, again with Dr. Sabin as the first author (which
you can again read for free here[iv]), makes the following intriguing
statements (again, emphasis is mine):

> "The second question at issue in hematology concerns
> the nature of the <u>stem cell</u>. It is accepted that there is a
> common stem cell for all the white blood cells. The only
> question at issue is whether this stem cell is identical
> with the lymphocyte or is a less differentiated type. It is
> clear that the stem cell is the lymphoidocyte of
> Pappenheim (22), or the lymphoid hemoblast of Jordan
> and Johnson (18). We have presented evidence for the
> theory that this cell, though it looks much like the small
> lymphocyte, <u>lacks certain signs of differentiation</u>."

This article is clearly focused on stem cells. Sabin even mentions that
the cells are undifferentiated, a key characteristic of stem cells. Sabin
also gives major credit to three scientists (Pappenheim as well as two
others) who came before her, placing her work in the appropriate

---

[iii]http://www.ncbi.nlm.nih.gov/pmc/articles/PMC2132174/pdf/267.pdf
[iv]http://www.ncbi.nlm.nih.gov/pmc/articles/PMC2133421/pdf/97.pdf

scientific context. I appreciate the fact that she did this as sometimes in science, including in the stem cell field, the process of crediting those who came earlier (and on whose shoulders we may be standing metaphorically speaking) falls through the cracks.

If one looks for the Pappenheim and Jordan & Johnson papers that Sabin cited we find that they were published earlier. Pappenheim's work includes that remarkable model of a stem cell tree (Figure 4.1) that I mentioned earlier.

Also notable is the work of Nobel Laureate E. Donnall Thomas[v] of the Hutch, who in the 1950s studied bone marrow transplantation. Thomas' research strongly supported the existence of hematopoietic stem cells as well even though they could not be sure at that time that stem cells were the driving force behind the success of the transplants. Thomas and his team discovered through work in dogs that there were specific cells in bone marrow that could restore hematopoiesis after lethal irradiation. For example, a 1957 article by Thomas, et al. in the prestigious *New England Journal of Medicine* clearly indicates the existence of special primitive bone marrow cells that can restore hematopoiesis [5].

Canadian scientists Drs. James Till and Ernset McCulloch also did pioneering studies in hematopoietic stem cell research. Their work deserves enormous credit. In my opinion one could easily argue that Till should already have a Nobel Prize (McCulloch passed away in 2011 and posthumous awards are not given). In 1963, Till and McCulloch published their seminal paper on hematopoietic stem cells in the journal *Nature*.

The title was the following: *Cytological demonstration of the clonal nature of spleen colonies derived from transplanted mouse marrow cells* [6]. Here is the first paragraph:

> "In normal mouse hæmatopoietic tissue, there is a class
> of cells which, on being transplanted into heavily
> irradiated mice, can proliferate and form macroscopic

---

[v]http://www.nobelprize.org/nobel_prizes/medicine/laureates/1990/

colonies. In the spleen, the colonies formed in this manner are discrete and easy to count. Microscopically, each colony appears as a cluster of hæmatopoiotic cells, many of which are dividing; and often, within a given colony, the cells which are observed indicate that differentiation is occurring along three lines, into cells of the erythrocytic, granulocytic and megakaryocytic series, respectively."

The colonies referred to in this passage consist of blood cells each generated from a hematopoietic stem cell. This was the first time that scientists had developed an assay to study stem cell function, a huge discovery. Still, I find it puzzling that Till and McCulloch did not employ the name "stem cells" even once in that paper since it was a well-established concept and nomenclature by that time in the hematology field. One year later they published a follow up study explicitly discussing that the colonies they observed came from stem cells.[vi] Their work profoundly changed and invigorated the stem cell field.

This brief history of stem cell research demonstrates that many researchers across the globe contributed to the discovery of stem cells and the work spanned more than a century. At some level, I would argue that the discovery of stem cells continues to this day.

Models of Stem Cells Based on Function

Overall, defining stem cells can be a complex task as mentioned earlier, but there are some fundamentals about stem cell functions that are particularly important for you to understand that I will outline below. And if we take a holistic approach considering many factors simultaneously we can confidently identify functional stem cells in most, even if not in all cases. The most effective way to understand stem cells is through models of how they behave. Just as Till and McCulloch developed a real functional assay or model in mice of hematopoietic stem cell function,

---

[vi]http://www.ncbi.nlm.nih.gov/pmc/articles/PMC300599/

scientists create models on paper and using computers to consider stem cells functions as well.

All stem cell functions are based on an intrinsic, unique adaptability they possess. In other words, stem cells are adept at taking on new cellular personalities. This flexibility in identity is called potency or "plasticity" and is at the heart of stem cell differentiation into a variety of other cell types. A stem cell might be a stem cell for a while, then be a progenitor for a certain period of time, and then cycle back to be a stem cell again. It is important to include this plasticity in our modeling of stem cell function.

In Pappenheim's model (Figure 4.1), the dominant stem cell is represented by the circle in the middle of the diagram connected to all the other cells (other circles) directly or indirectly by lines and arrows. In Figure 4.2, I present my own simplified stem cell fate tree that is less elegant than Pappenheim's, but intended to be more intuitive. My goal in this model in Figure 4.2 is that you easily can identify and learn the types of cells and concepts and then apply them to the complex model in Figure 4.1 from more than a hundred years ago.

My model shows stem cells on the left in the niche (the home of stem cells, discussed in more depth in the next chapter). As they divide they can differentiate (showing their potency) or self-renewal to produce more stem cells. This model also illustrates an important concept for you to know related to the two types of stem cell division: symmetric and asymmetric. When stem cells undergo symmetric division they produce two daughter cells that are also stem cells, but when asymmetric division occurs one daughter cell is a stem cell and one is a more limited cell (e.g. a progenitor) destined to produce differentiated cells.

Exactly how stem cells maintain the flexibility to change their identities is not entirely understood, but a major factor is their epigenome (discussed in more depth in the previous chapter). In the 1950s, a biologist named Dr. Hal Waddington conceived of a topological landscape as a model of stem cell fate linked to epigenetics and the epigenome (the elements that control DNA structure and hence activity) [7].

Stem cell fate tree

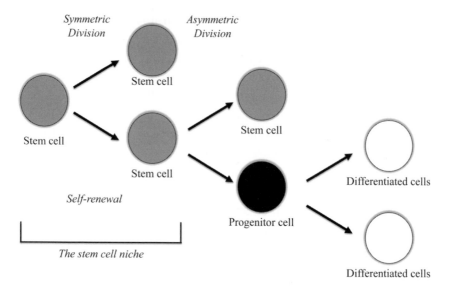

Figure 4.2. Hypothetical stem cell fate tree model. Gray cells are stem cells, the black cell is a progenitor cell, and white cells are differentiated cells. The stem cell niche (discussed in depth in the next chapter), home of stem cells, would be on the left side of the diagram spatially.

In the Waddington model, the top of the model was "higher" and cells there possessed more of a cellular energy in a sense. The most stem-like cells are at the top and more differentiated cells are at the bottom. In one way of thinking, the Waddington model is akin to a cell fate tree such as mine in Figure 4.2 and Pappenheim's in Figure 4.1, but in three dimensions. As cells roll down the hill in channels they take on more defined fates based on epigenetic changes. In such a model the level of "stemness" decreases as cells roll down the hill. Incorporating our increasing realization of the plasticity of stem cells, new Waddington-inspired models have been made to include variable cell fates and iPS cells.

Figure 4.3 is my own Waddington-inspired model brought to life via a collaborative effort with scientific illustrator Taylor Seamount, an intern in my lab and updated to include new concepts. The model not only incorporates differentiation, but also cell death, reprogramming (the cell being pulled back up the hill) to make iPS cells, and cancer formation as well. In this model the stem cell niche would be at the top. Differentiated cells are at the bottom.

Even amongst stem cells there is variety as there are dozens of kinds, but they fall into three main groups. Some are **multipotent**, meaning they are able to self-renewal and can also make multiple types of differentiated cells (hence multipotent). Multipotent stem cells are the most common kind of stem cell in the body and a good example of multipotent stem cells are hematopoietic (or blood forming) stem cells.

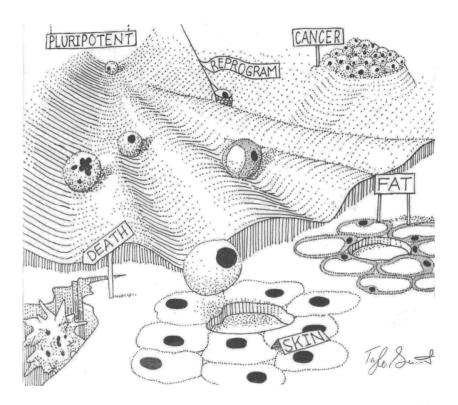

Figure 4.3. A Waddington-inspired model topographical landscape of cellular plasticity and fate by the author and Taylor Seamount.

Pluripotent stem cells can make any type of cell in the human body except extraembryonic tissues such as specific parts of the placenta (hence the term pluripotent with "pluri" meaning multiple or more). Pluripotent stem cells include embryonic stem cells and iPS cells. The different types of pluripotent stem cells were discussed in more depth, intercompared, and compared to adult stem cells in Chapter 2. **Totipotent** stem cells also exist but there is only one kind: the fertilized egg (also called a zygote). It can form every type of human cell including extraembryonic ones (hence the name "totipotent".)

In Waddington's model and in adaptations such as mine, the more potent the stem cell, the higher up on the landscape it resides. As a result, pluripotent cells are at the top. Cells rolling down the hill might be multipotent stem cells or progenitor cells. Cells at the bottom are differentiated cells. When differentiated cells are reprogrammed such as during iPS cell formation, they must (in our model) be dragged back up the hill to a pluripotent state. That "dragging" process involves the epigenetic factors such as Oct4, Sox2, Klf4, and c-Myc, which drive the cell back up the slope to a pluripotent state.

On my model landscape of cell fate, cells can also go astray. For example, stem cells may acquire mutations or epigenomic glitches and end up off on the "wrong path" leading to cancer formation. Sometimes cells also are damaged in ways to lead to their death. I appreciate models that include not just good, but also real potential bad outcomes because they help us to understand how those events occur and potentially prevent them.

A New Global Symbol for Stem Cells for the Future

Another kind of model is a symbol. Surprisingly to my knowledge there is no global symbol for stem cells of any kind in the world. Therefore, I am proposing here a new global symbol for stem cells inspired by the cell fate tree models that we have been discussing.

In this new symbol (Figure 4.4), which can also be thought of as a model of sorts in the shape of a tree, I have tried to convey the ability of one stem cell to make a rainbow of differentiated cell types. Hence, the stem cell (at the bottom in the trunk of the tree) is depicted as a rainbow cell and as we go up the tree and out on branches, cells become less stem-like and more differentiated as reflected by their different colors.

My hope with this symbol is that it resonates with people all around the world, many of whom may not speak English. For this reason I have incorporated the "trunk" concept that is integral to the idea and language of stem cells in other languages (see below), in which they have named stem cells "trunk cells". <u>As you have seen from the history of the discovery of stem cells, stem cell research and the importance for stem cells as medicine are truly global issues.</u>

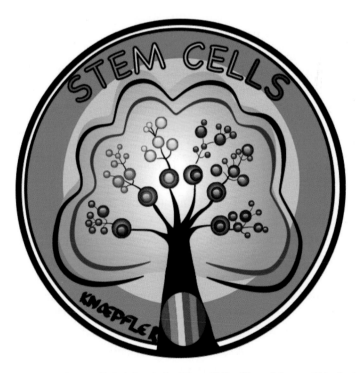

Figure 4.4. Proposed New Global Symbol of Stem Cells. The rainbow cell in the trunk of the symbolic tree is the multipotent stem cell.

Not Lost in Translation: A Global Model of Stem Cells for the Future

One of my blog's mottos is "stem cells not lost in translation".

What do I mean?

"Stem cells" is one of those terms we use quite often without thinking about it. But why do we (in English and many other languages) call them "stem cells"?

The name "stem" would appear to be a reflection of their multi- or pluripotent nature. The term "stem" in this case refers to the stem of a plant meaning that stem cells have the potential to branch down different pathways and support growth. I am sure "stem" is used in addition because of its alternate meaning of something from which other things originate.

But why do we not call "stem" cells something else?

Could there be a better name than "stem" cells?

Other languages provide some helpful lessons here.

Interestingly, in both Portuguese and Chinese, "stem cell" is translated literally as "trunk cell". This is appropriate as it gives the same kind of meaning as "stem" cell in the plant/tree kind of sense, but I think "trunk cell" (at least in English) actually makes more sense than "stem cell" because from a trunk grows the entire rest of the tree including many branches, leaves, flowers, etc. In contrast, sometimes from a plant stem there is just a flower or a leaf.

In Spanish, "stem cell" is translated as "mother cell". The term "mother cell" also makes good sense to me because it suggests that the stem cell can give rise to daughter cells. Note that for whatever reason in the stem cell research field we call the cells that are produced from a stem cell "daughter cells" and not "son cells". The original cell that divides is called either the "parental" or "mother" cell, not father cell.

In Albanian, "stem cell" is translated as "flow cell". This is intriguing and suggests to me a flowing river that can go down different paths.

In both Turkish and Azerbaijani, "stem cell" is "root cell". I think root might be a better term than stem.

In Vietnamese, "stem cell" is "original cell".

In Croatian, "stem cell" is "home cell".

In Welsh, "stem cell" is "basic cell".

To summarize, the words used instead of stem in other languages include the following: trunk, mother, flow, root, original, home, and basic.

I like all of them and they all have interesting connotations.

I think "trunk cell" sounds the most interesting, but I imagine we will not see a change in nomenclature any time soon in English. Besides some folks might get confused and think a trunk cell is from an elephant. I should note that many languages translate "stem cell" as just "stem cell" as it is in English.

The Cultural Language of Stem Cells

Just as there are many ways of saying "stem cells" around the world, there are also a host of different beliefs about stem cells. For example, notions about embryonic stem cell research and the question of when life begins (issues discussed in depth in Chapter 12) vary dramatically in different countries and cultures. This diversity of perspectives is refreshing to me. I believe we need to avoid the trap of ethnocentrism when it comes to stem cells and embrace the reality that people have very different views.

There is an interesting article from Joy Resmovits in *Forward* that compares attitudes about and funding for embryonic stem cell research in Israel and in the US.[vii] In the article, Resmovits discusses how in contrast to the US where there is divisive debate in this area that slows research, in Israel the government and public more broadly and actively support such research. The end result is that per capita, Israel is 10 times more productive than the US in this research area.

She also points out that in Judaism, life does not begin until at least 40 days after conception, making the few-day old blastocysts used to produce embryonic stem cells merely IVF-derived clusters of a few dozen simply cells and not human beings. Interestingly, in Islam and other religions human life also is commonly not thought to occur at

---

[vii]http://forward.com/articles/134819/two-countries-two-approaches-to-regulating-embryon/

conception, but later. Although even amongst practitioners of any single religion I am sure there is a range of opinions. The bottom line is that there is a diversity not only of stem cell nomenclatures in the languages of the world, but also in views about stem cells.

References

1. Ramalho-Santos M, Willenbring H: **On the origin of the term "stem cell".** *Cell Stem Cell* 2007, **1:**35-38.
2. Pappenheim A: *Atlas der menschlichen blutzellen.* Jena,: G. Fischer; 1905.
3. Arrick MS: **Stem cell lymphoma of the newborn.** *Archives of pathology* 1946, **42:**104-110.
4. Sabin FR, Doan CA, Forkner CE: **The Production of Osteogenic Sarcomata and the Effects on Lymph Nodes and Bone Marrow of Intravenous Injections of Radium Chloride and Mesothorium in Rabbits.** *The Journal of experimental medicine* 1932, **56:**267-289.
5. Thomas ED, Lochte HL, Jr., Lu WC, Ferrebee JW: **Intravenous infusion of bone marrow in patients receiving radiation and chemotherapy.** *N Engl J Med* 1957, **257:**491-496.
6. Becker AJ, Mc CE, Till JE: **Cytological demonstration of the clonal nature of spleen colonies derived from transplanted mouse marrow cells.** *Nature* 1963, **197:**452-454.
7. Waddington CH: *The strategy of the genes; a discussion of some aspects of theoretical biology.* New York,: Macmillan; 1957.

Chapter 5

All in the Family: An Insider's Tale of Two Stem Cells and a Black Sheep

In this chapter I take you for a virtual tour inside both of a stem cell lab and a prototypic stem cell itself. I also go through a typical day in the cellular lives of three key types of stem cells: an endogenous stem cell, a laboratory grown stem cell, and the black sheep of the family, a cancer stem cell. Together this "family" of stem cells (Figure 5.1) has a lot to teach us about the stem cell field.

Starting the Tour: A Backstage Pass to a Stem Cell Lab

Ever wonder what goes on in a stem cell research lab? How does a lab function to produce that cutting-edge research that you read about? What are the main concerns of the scientists handling the stem cells and doing the experiments? Who are they? What is a lab really like? In this chapter I will start by giving you an insider's tour of a stem cell lab.

A clear understanding of how a stem cell lab works and is run will be fundamental to your overall understanding of stem cells including their therapeutic application.

Stem cell labs come in two main types.

First and most common is the stem cell research laboratory where mostly basic, but also sometimes translational research occurs.

The second type of lab is a clinical production lab, sometimes referred to as a GMP (Good Manufacturing Practices) lab, where stem cell products are produced that are of the appropriate quality that they can be transplanted into human patients with FDA approval. My main focus in this chapter is on the former type of stem cell lab where more basic, pre-clinical research is conducted.

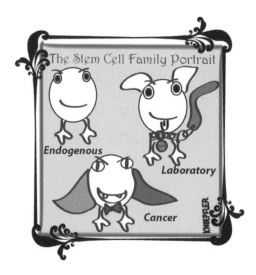

Figure 5.1. The three stem cell types discussed in this Chapter: (an endogenous) stem cell, a laboratory (akin to a domesticated pet) stem cell, and cancer stem cell portrayed as a family.

However, first I want to go over the key elements of a GMP lab. In contrast to a research lab, a GMP lab has to meet strict specifications in a number of ways to keep the stem cell products that are produced pathogen-free. For example, airflow is quite crucial in a GMP lab and must be directed in specific ways to keep unfiltered outside air from entering the lab where it could contaminate cells. Typically GMP personnel must shower as well as change into sterile clothing and protective outfits as well. All the growth media and other materials in a GMP lab must be sterile both inside and out of the bottles or containers. GMP labs must keep strict records on all these and other issues as well. If you think this sounds expensive and complicated, you are right, but it is crucial to protect patients.

Disturbingly, instead, many for-profit stem cell clinics use stem cell research quality lab setups to produce stem cell products that are then transplanted into patients. As a cost-saving measure, they bypass the expense of creating and maintaining the necessary GMP lab that would protect patient safety far more rigorously.

What is a stem cell research lab like and how does it operate?

A typical stem cell research lab has a somewhat hierarchical structure. Running the lab is a person called a principal investigator or "PI". The PI has a very frenetic job that some might say is multi-tasking taken to an extreme. Responsibilities include fund raising (writing grants, contacting foundations, and so forth), public relations (giving seminars, traveling to meetings, and increasingly engaging in social media), service such as being on committees (if in academia), teaching, and supervising all aspects of their research laboratory. The last item is in itself an umbrella job encompassing many things including experimental design, data interpretation, paper writing, teaching in the lab, and working with trainees (undergraduates, graduate students, postdocs, medical students) and technicians. As a PI myself, I love the job.

Depending on the size of the research lab, many have an employee who acts as the lab manager. In some cases this is a Ph.D. level scientist with many years of postdoctoral experience. Other times the lab manager is a senior technician who manages the day-to-day running of lab including such things as ordering supplies, compliance with institutional regulations, training, and so forth. However, ultimately the PI is responsible for all of these things, especially should something go wrong.

Within the hierarchy of a lab, the next level is usually for postdoctoral fellows, colloquially called "postdocs". Generally, postdocs are scientists who have received a Ph.D. (or M.D. less commonly). They are receiving additional training and experience prior to either attempting to find their own job as a PI or moving on to other work such as in industry, science writing, teaching, and the like. Very large labs, of which there are many in the stem cell field, are often highly populated by postdocs at least in part because postdocs can in theory obtain their own funding through fellowships and other sources.

Graduate students working in stem cell research must do years of doctoral work prior to receiving their Ph.D. Being less experienced, they typically require more oversight by the PI, although it is a PI's job to mentor both postdocs and students in their labs. Many labs, including my own also have undergraduate students getting research experience. Obtaining funding is far more difficult for undergraduate and graduate students by comparison to postdocs.

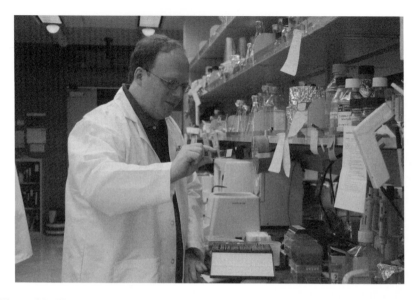

Figure 5.2. The author examining a slide in his research lab at UC Davis School of Medicine.

An integral part of the lab routine of most labs is something we refer to as "lab meeting" at which people in the lab take turns presenting their work. Weekly lab meetings are a good opportunity to brain storm and discuss particular roadblocks or reasons for excitement. Lab meetings are one of my favorite events of the week and do not involve fighting.

Research labs are busy places full of equipment and activity (see mine in Figure 5.2). After all these years, my lab is like a second home for me.

An Insider's Tour of a Prototypic Stem Cell

The stem cell membrane

Now that we have toured a lab, I will take a virtual tour of a stem cell itself. I want you to turn up your creativity and imagine we have adjusted the scale of the world such that you are the size of an ant and a stem cell is the size of a tennis ball. From this perspective we can get a close look at the most vital parts of stem cells. Before you walk with me inside of our virtual stem cell, we will survey the outside.

From the exterior, this stem cell looks akin to a tennis ball, but not quite so round. It contains a fuzz of proteins on the outside attached to its cell membrane. The cell membrane is equivalent to our skin in some ways. For example, it in part protects the cell from the outside world and holds it together. Some of the cell membrane-associated proteins are part of the cell's protein identity code that we talked about in the immunity section earlier in the book. Other proteins on the membrane of a stem cell are called "receptors" that allow the cell to sense and respond to its environmental conditions such as the levels of growth factors.

From the outside, our stem cell's appearance looks in almost every respect indistinguishable from many non-stem cells. However, the nature of that protein fuzz on the cell membrane of stem cells is quite different from that of non-stem cells, allowing the cells to respond to the same environment differently. For example, many stem cells have an abundance of receptors for the growth factor FGF, but also for other kinds of growth factors. The exact overall collection of these receptors is unique in stem cells.

Going through the membrane into the cytoplasm

Now as we step through the outer cellular membrane on our way into the cytoplasm (the "body" of the cell), we turn on our headlamp like a miner. We can see the membrane in cross-section as we squeeze through it. You observe that some of the proteins making up that fuzz on the cell membrane are long and skinny, and many are not just on the outside of the cell. Quite a few of these proteins extend from the outside of the cell all the way through the membrane and into the inside of the cell. Therefore, it is not surprising that they as a group are called "transmembrane" proteins. They are the only proteins in cells that are both on the outside of the cell and simultaneously on the inside. As a result, they are uniquely positioned to transmit information from the outside of the cell to the inside. For example, when two cells touch, transmembrane proteins "feel" that and send signals inside the cell to stimulate a response.

Growth factors and their matching receptors on the cell membrane bind each other through a lock-and-key like mechanism. When lock and key fit together, a signal is triggered inside the cell influencing cell behavior. If they do not precisely fit together, there is no signal. Overall, the cell membrane is not only what protects the cell from the outside world, but also it is the main way in which cells communicate with that external universe including other cells.

The surprisingly powerful stem cell cytoplasm

We continue our cellular tour, passing through the membrane (sort of akin to a border crossing) we can see that there are differences in the patterns and types of transmembrane receptors in stem cells versus non-stem cells. This unique membrane protein signature of stem cells makes them respond to the outside world in a unique way. It is through this type of communication that stem cells can be told by other cells (a process called "paracrine" signaling, which means signaling between two different cells) or even tell themselves ("autocrine" signaling) to do certain things.

A specific signal may tell a stem cell to continue on in its cellular life as a stem cell or instead to differentiate into a specific type of specialized cell such as a beating heart cell. Autocrine growth factor signaling in stem cells might reasonably be compared to the cell giving itself a pat on the back or alternatively under certain circumstances, convincing itself to commit suicide.

Now that we are through the membrane we have made it into the cytoplasm, the "guts" of the cell. The cytoplasm of cells is aqueous, but so full of proteins and other large molecules that the texture is more akin to a thick gel than water. Much the same as our "guts" have organs, the cytoplasm of the cell has organelles (meaning "little organs") that have specific jobs.

Inside the cytoplasm of our stem cell, again most of what we see is cellular machinery and organelles that appears much the same as other cells. Yet there are differences in the levels and compositions of specific

RNAs and proteins in the stem cell cytoplasm versus that of a non-stem cell. Certain RNAs and proteins are quite stem cell specific and help that stem cell to keep its identity.

Interesting nuclear transfer experiments, in which nuclei are transferred from a non-stem cell into an oocyte (egg cell) that had its own nucleus removed (a process called "enucleation"), indicate that the oocyte cytoplasm is quite powerful. These studies showed conclusively that just the cytoplasm of an oocyte could reprogram the transferred nucleus of a non-stem cell to make it behave essentially identically to a nucleus of an oocyte. This is another form of cellular reprogramming akin to making iPS cells. Nuclear transfer is also the basis of cloning, discussed further from ethical and technical perspectives in Chapter 12.

Getting to the heart of the matter: The nucleus

Now if we step inside the nucleus of the stem cell we see chromatin, which is the DNA of the cell wrapped up and packaged with a bunch of proteins including most importantly transcription factors and specific DNA binding proteins including histones that are part of the epigenome discussed in Chapter 3.

In the stem cell nucleus there are distinct features of the stem cell. Stem cell chromatin is packaged such that some regions of DNA are actively made into RNA and translated into proteins in ways that simply do not occur in non-stem cells. Other regions of the DNA including certain genes in stem cells are packaged so tightly that no RNA or protein can be made from them. Some of these are differentiation-associated genes that make proteins that tell specialized cells to do their jobs. Stem cells do not make such proteins unless signaled to differentiate.

Scientists use the unique features of the stem cell membrane, cytoplasm, and nucleus as a means of identifying stem cells via specific technologies that will be discussed more in future chapters.

Step back outside the stem cell and imagine it is in its native context. You will see that it does not live inside a vacuum or in isolation, but rather in a very special place in tissues called the "niche" (pronounced "nee-shh"). In the niche, the stem cell is surrounded by other cells and a gooey substance secreted by cells called "extracellular matrix", which is basically a thick, viscous couch of proteins and other factors. This matrix keeps stem cells, which sit on and sink into it, very cozy and happy. A stem cell in its niche is like a coach potato.

Our next goal in this chapter is to compare typical days in the lives of endogenous and laboratory stem cells as well as cancer stem cells. It is worth noting that only an endogenous stem cell has a normal, cozy niche and laboratory cells must get by without a true niche relying on a fake one. Various methods are employed by stem cell scientists to keep our laboratory stem cells, which we consider almost like pets or lab mascots, as happy as possible living on plastic dishes in incubators.

I will begin our comparison of different types of stem cells by describing a typical day for an endogenous stem cell living in our body and the role of the niche.

A Day in the Cellular Life of an Endogenous Stem Cell

While the different types of endogenous stem cells vary in their functions and characteristics depending on the organ or tissue in which they reside, there are many common themes. For example, while a hematopoietic stem cell of the blood system and a stem cell living in muscle have many distinctions, in a number of critical ways they are quite similar. A dependency on the niche is just one example. What is the niche?

The niche

Stem cells by and large are very sensitive cells that require the specific environment (which we in science call the "microenvironment" simply because it is really small) of the niche in which to live in order for them to remain stem cells. In real estate and businesses such as restaurants, the mantra is "location, location, location". For stem cells one should apply the same saying.

A cell's identity is strongly influenced by its neighborhood. Take a normal stem cell out of its niche and it will have a very difficult if not impossible time maintaining its "stemness" or stem cell-like nature over time.

What constitutes a stem cell niche?

The stem cell niches of different organs can have some variability in terms of design and components, but generally the niches exist in relatively protected areas of the body. They also share four key elements that operate together to maintain stem cell identity: (1) an entourage of neighboring cells, (2) a specific type of extracellular matrix (that cellular glue or stew mentioned above that holds cells together and in which they sit, but that also greatly influences their identity and behavior), (3) a "soup" of growth factors and cytokines provided in a liquid in which the cells are bathed, and (4) a specialized physical environment consisting of various factors such as pH, oxygen tension, pressure, and so forth. Together these four elements are what actively keep a stem cell in possession of its stemness.

Niche neighbors

In a typical day for an endogenous stem cell in the niche, its neighboring cells hug it, communicate with it (via growth factors that use the lock-and-key mechanism on the cell membrane to trigger signals inside the cell), and support its stem cell-related properties. By analogy, one might imagine a stem cell as a rock star surrounded by his supportive entourage, limos, mansion, and so forth. As much as cells can operate in a "cell-autonomous" (meaning independent of external factors) fashion, the neighboring cells in the niche influence to a great extent how stem cells behave. For example, niche neighbors influence the likelihood of a stem cell to stay in the niche or exit to perform some specific function or turn into a differentiated cell, one-way trips from which the stem cell will likely never return. The niche neighbors to a large extent decide the stem cell's fate: to be or not to be a stem cell.

Extracellular matrix

Stem cells also live within a thick stew of proteins that not only "talk" to the cell and provide it instructions, but also support the stem cell physically. Imagine eggs in a carton; the extracellular matrix is the carton for the stem cells in the body. However, the relationship between the cell and extracellular matrix is far more intimate than that. The cell and the matrix are continuous so that where the cell membrane ends and the matrix begins may not always be obvious in the native context. The matrix of the stem cell niche is unique and particularly supportive of stem cells.

Growth factors

Stem cells are, as discussed earlier, coated with receptors on their outer membranes that sense other cells and the levels of growth factors in the surrounding environment. These growth factors can come from neighboring cells, the matrix, the blood stream, or even the stem cell itself. The collective concentrations and diversity of growth factors that the stem cell senses have a powerful influence on its behavior and fate.

Physical environment

Scientists are learning more and more about how influential the physical environment (oxygen tension, pH, temperature, pressure, etc.) of the niche is on stem cells. For decades scientists have been happy if the stem cells they had in the lab would just grow under laboratory conditions (more on that below in our discussion of a day in the life of a laboratory cell). Now, however, researchers are striving to make the laboratory physical conditions as similar to those of the niche as possible. It is a difficult challenge given the complexity of the endogenous niche.

Leaving the niche

A key principle to introduce here is that the default state of stem cells is surprisingly not to stay a stem cell, but rather to differentiate. The principle that stem cells will turn into a non-stem cell unless actively told otherwise appears to be true of most types of stem cells. Stem cells essentially are designed to differentiate into a specialized non-stem cell type in most environments outside the niche. Therefore, cells and tissues must actively and cooperatively maintain a stem cell state by opposing default forces that promote differentiation. A general rule of thumb is that as stem cells move (yes, cells in your body including stem cells frequently do crawl around), the greater the distance that they are from the stem cell niche, the less stem-like they tend to become.

Imagine you are about to go on a journey away from home, a place that you have lived all of your life, for the first time. And you are never coming back. As you travel and time passes while you are away from home, you spend your life in other countries. You begin to speak other languages and take on other customs. You eat the foods of other countries. Literally who you are begins to change because of the environmental influence on you. By analogy, for stem cells, their home is almost always the niche. The further removed they are from it and the longer that time passes away, the more likely they are to take on a new identity that is no longer stem-like.

If an endogenous stem cell is to become a differentiated cell, a critical question is what type. For example, certain stem cells such as MSCs that we have discussed earlier can become any of a number of types of cells: bone, cartilage, blood vessels, adipose (fat), and perhaps others as well. A neural stem cell can become neurons or other brain cell types called astrocytes and oligodendrocytes.

The new, differentiated cell identity for the former stem cell is to a large extent controlled by its new non-niche environment, but also sometimes by other cells in the niche that in a sense perhaps give the stem cells a metaphorical push in the direction of a certain fate.

Extending our earlier traveler analogy further, if a person leaves England and spends the rest of their life in Brazil (because their parents, akin to niche neighbors bought them tickets to Rio) they will become one kind of person, whereas if the same person spends the rest of their life in India, they will be quite different. In both scenarios, they are truly less English than before they left home, but the changes are very different in each case. The same is true of stem cells in that after they leave their niche, the characteristics of their new tissue home will greatly influence what type of cell they become.

On any given day, an endogenous stem cell might receive signals from the environment leading to its mobilization to leave the niche or alternatively to its retention in the niche. Most often in healthy people the latter signaling, to stay put in the niche, predominates for the vast majority of stem cells. Mobilization signals (similar to a person receiving a draft notice to enter the military during war time and report to a certain new place, or your parents kicking you out of their home after getting fed up), when they do come, might indicate that there has been an injury or that a certain cellular population has reached a lower threshold where action by the stem cell is needed. However, most stem cells simply stay ensconced in the niche, protected from a wide variety of potential cellular insults. A stem cell may reside in this manner for years or even decades depending on the tissue and health of the person in which it resides.

If a stem cell does leave the niche, most likely there is no coming back. That exit is fateful, as the cell will ultimately differentiate, proliferate to form progenitor cells, or die. Only rarely will a stem cell leave the niche, travel elsewhere in the body, and then return and remain a stem cell. Generally, with the most prominent exception of stem cells of the blood (hematopoietic stem cells), stem cells that are on the move within given tissues do not travel far, most likely less than 1mm. Thus, for example, an endogenous stem cell in abdominal fat, most likely an MSC, will never go to the face or into a joint. There is a reason for this restriction in stem cell travel as their functions in most cases are location-specific.

Yet, some doctors are charging patients tens of thousands of dollars to remove adipose or fat-derived stem cells from abdominal fat (via liposuction) and transplant the cells into faces, joints, and many other places in the body. Whether these displaced laboratory stem cells will behave properly and do what the doctors intend in their new home remains largely unknown.

It is also thought that even stem cells that are called by the same name such as "fat stem cells" are different depending on their anatomic location. For example, abdominal fat as a tissue is functionally different than facial fat, and their respective populations of fat stem cells are different as well. These differences increase the risks that transfer of fat stem cells from one part of the body to another could lead to unintended consequences. I will discuss this risk further in the next section of this chapter on laboratory grown stem cells.

Even within the relative safety of the niche, endogenous stem cells can meet untimely fates. For example, if an endogenous stem cell is unfortunate enough to acquire specific mutations in its DNA, it may either trigger its own death via apoptosis or potentially take the first step toward becoming a cancer stem cell, with the former far more likely.

Over time, the number of endogenous stem cells we each possess as adults tends to go down with age and as I describe in the next chapter, I have proposed a new theory of aging in which the lower the number of healthy endogenous stem cells that we each possess, the faster we age.

My Pet Stem Cell: The Very Different Cellular Life in a Lab

How are laboratory stem cells different than endogenous?

I have a pet stem cell in my lab that might fill you in on the answer to this question.

Actually I do not, but many times it feels that way.

In the research lab setting, caring for stem cells is not that different in many ways than having a needy pet. I am going to build on that analogy in this section to help you understand how different cellular life is for a stem cell in a lab versus an endogenous stem cell as well as just how challenging that care of stem cells can be.

Growing stem cells is neither easy nor cheap. Unlike the personal computer revolution, revolutionary stem cell research going on today cannot be done in the family garage growing stem cells using Tupperware™ and a microwave leading to some breakthrough. Stem cell technology is fundamentally different than other types of cutting edge technology. While computer or Internet startups could indeed germinate in one's parents' garage, to do something like that with stem cells you would have to build a lab in your garage likely costing $100,000 or more even if you bought your equipment on E-bay. State and federal regulators are likely to frown on this DIY garage human stem cell lab as well, potentially throwing you in jail.

But if stem cells were domesticated and you brought them into your home, I think you would view them as something akin to the most spoiled, expensive pets in the world, and then they probably would die on you like the proverbial dead gold fish that your dad flushes down the drain.

We can learn a great deal about stem cells by thinking of them as "pets" and the decision making process that goes into deciding whether to get a pet. In fact, my family was thinking of getting a dog a few years back. Our three daughters had been asking for one for years. I have generally sided with them, while my wife is the formidable force opposing us. She played the devil's advocate by asking incisive, but very smart questions.

Who will feed the dog and what will they feed dog?
Who will clean up after the dog?
Who will take the dog for walks?
Where is the dog going to sleep?
Who will take care of the dog when we are on vacation?
How will you know if the dog is sick and who will take it to the vet?
What will we name the dog?
What exactly will we get out of having this dog?

I thought our answers to these questions were usually not very convincing to my wife, but in the end we did end up getting a dog, a female black lab named "Elvis" that came with that name when we got her. At least we did not have to fuss over her name.

For better or worse, in my research lab and that of other stem cell scientists, stem cells are kind of like our pets. But unfortunately they are extraordinarily high-maintenance pets, and now that we have them in my lab, in retrospect, perhaps I should have asked the same questions about them as I listed above for my family's dog Elvis before we adopted her.

Who is going to feed the stem cells and what are they going to feed them?
Who will clean up after the stem cells?
Who will take the stem cells for walks?
Where are the stem cells going to sleep?
Who will take care of our stem cells when we go on vacation?
How will you know if the stem cells are sick and what will you do about it?

What will we name the stem cells?

What exactly will we get out of having these stem cells?

Let us imagine that stem cells are laboratory pets for a moment. The answers to each of these questions will teach you a great deal about laboratory stem cells and how we do research on them.

Who is going to feed the stem cells and what are they going to feed them?

Stem cell scientists do need to feed laboratory stem cells and the cells do eat in their own way as alluded to in previous chapters. Their food is based on a liquid that we in the stem cell field call "media" or "medium" (singular). Stem cell medium is akin to a nutrient rich KoolAid™ both in appearance and content.

While I can open up a bag of dog chow, dump it into the bowl for Elvis, and that will do the trick (even though she is somewhat fussy compared to other dogs), the fussiness of stem cells about their food has no parallel.

Their food has to be ultra clean, in fact sterile, and they only are happy with the most expensive ingredients. Their stem cell "chow" must also be warm, ideally precisely 98.6 degrees, and not too sour (pH) or sweet (glucose). Because stem cells are prone to infection, we always spike their food with antibiotics as well. Stem cells are akin to an unfortunate little kid with ear infections for two years who has to choke down penicillin every day in pink liquid. We also frequently spike the stem cell medium with high concentrations of the pricey (approximately $1 billion/lb.) growth factor FGF, which the stem cells gobble up quickly. Fortunately cells only "eat" billionths of a pound of FGF, but a stem cell lab can still spend a fortune on it.

For all these reasons, liquid stem cell chow ends up being literally more expensive than the fanciest French Champagne. And the stem cells, well, they have a drinking problem so the stuff often must be replaced with fresh chow.

The question of who is going to feed the stem cells their stem cell chow is tougher than you might think. Stem cells are hungry little beasties and turn up their noses at food that is more than a day or so old.

As a result, in many cases they must be fed every day, 365 days a year including weekends and holidays, which can make their keepers, us scientists, very grouchy.

The overall objective of how we feed stem cells is to recapitulate aspects of the stem cell niche including growth factors, small molecules, and so forth discussed in the previous chapter.

As you can see, feeding stem cells is not a simple matter and despite our best efforts the laboratory stem cells at some level know they are in a fake niche so they do not function quite the same as endogenous stem cells.

Friends without benefits: Feeder cells

Another way we indirectly feed stem cells is using other cells as the suppliers of growth factors and additional substances. Stem cells do not like to be alone and as mentioned earlier, a key element of the endogenous stem cell niche are other cells that keep stem cells happy and healthy. In the stem cell lab, where we grow the cells without a proper niche, we pay for little cellular friends to keep our stem cells company. Typically these are called "feeder cells".

Prior to adding our stem cells to a plastic dish to try to grow them, often times we first add a whole bunch of feeder cells that together form a "feeder layer" that covers the plastic. When we later add our stem cells they live on or snuggled up next to the feeder layer cells. Feeder layer cells were given that name as they not only physically support the stem cells, but also because they "feed" them. Feeder cells secrete growth factors that the stem cells drink up from the media, but also as feeder and stem cells physically touch, it is thought that the feeder cells may directly place proteins including growth factors onto the surface of stem cells. Feeder cells also secrete extracellular matrix for the stem cells that has similarities to the matrix found in the niche.

What exactly are the feeder cells and where do they come from? The type of feeder cell depends on which variety of stem cells one is growing in the lab. For embryonic stem cells and iPS cells, feeder layers are composed of fibroblasts, usually a type called "mouse embryonic fibroblasts" or MEFs for short. MEFs are used as feeder layer cells because scientists have empirically determined that pluripotent stem cells grow happily on MEFs. An example of this can be seen in Figure 2.2, where the feeders MEFs appear on the sides of an embryonic stem cell colony as spindle-shaped cells.

Immediately prior to using MEFs as feeder cells, scientists typically half-kill the MEFs first using either radiation or chemicals. The resulting zombie MEFs still produce lots of growth factors and other desirable proteins such as those of the extracellular matrix, which stem cells find highly beneficial. However, the zombie MEFs cannot proliferate at all. This cellular infertility of a sorts is an essential feature of feeder cells because it means that in a culture of stem cells living on top of feeder cells, only the stem cells will grow. As a result the MEFs do not have a chance to compete with the stem cells. In some ways the MEFs are similar to court eunuchs of olden days who were castrated and MEF lives are akin to the eunuch lives as servants to royalty with whom they lived, but could not couple with or marry. As a result, the feeder MEFs get no benefits out of serving the stem cells.

Stem cell scientists are largely happy with feeder cells because they make stem cells grow well in a dish in the lab. However, feeder cells are expensive and it is a hassle to have to continually turn them into cellular zombies. More significantly, it remains unclear how laboratory stem cells might be different from endogenous ones because feeder cells are not quite the same as the niche neighboring cells in the body. For clinical use, labs need to avoid the use of MEFs (which are difficult to separate entirely from the human stem cells and contaminate the human stem cells with mouse proteins that can trigger immune reactions in patients). Instead, such labs are increasingly depending on special, extra-expensive media that makes stem cell grow without a feeder layer.

Who will clean up after the stem cells?

You may be happy to know that unlike a dog who may leave you a "present" in any number of places from your bed, favorite chair, or rose bed to the new carpet, stem cells do not pee or poop, at least not that you can see or smell. Thank goodness. However, when you work with human stem cells especially, you might think they were pooping and peeing up a storm, because everything that comes in contact with them as well as their stem cell chow, is officially classified as biohazardous waste. As a result we go through a very large number of those red bags with the large frightening biohazardous symbol that you see on the TV show *CSI* that contain body parts.

When we care for our stem cells we also have to wear gloves, a lab coat, and goggles. We are not only protecting the stem cells from pathogens that we carry around with us, but also shielding ourselves from viruses or other nasties that the stem cells may contain that could infect us, particularly if the stem cells are human in origin. In addition, stem cells do secrete wastes into their media including metabolites.

Who will take the stem cell for walks?

My dog Elvis has a lot of energy and needs at least two walks a day. Luckily stem cells do not like to go for walks as we think of it with pets even if they do slowly crawl around in their dishes as they do inside the human body naturally, but unfortunately we have to take them places anyway to study them.

Sometimes these field trips do not go well.

Taking stem cells out of their incubators is risky business. They are sensitive to just about everything, especially temperature and air as well as germs. As a result, when we take them out for a "walk" to study them, we always figuratively and sometimes literally hold our breath.

If only you could put a leash on stem cells and lead them around that would be easier than what scientists have to do to move stem cells. We really only have two options. The first, for long distances, would be similar to cryogenically preserving your dog, flying her cross country in liquid nitrogen, and then thawing her at her new home. Sound stressful? For dogs it would not yield too many survivors either.

For stem cells, we put them in their "crate" (cryotube), freeze them in a special solution, and ship them off around the globe. They usually do pretty well on the journey and defrost better than most frozen waffles, but not always. Sometimes they are dead on arrival.

The other way to take stem cells for a walk (literally in this case), which we often need to do to conduct experiments on them, is in a little dish full of their liquid stem cell chow as we trot down the hall to specific equipment. For example, we do this in order to look at them on a special microscope or to sort them into different subpopulations using a fancy technique called "flow cytometry" that I will discuss in more detail later on in this chapter.

It is tricky, though, to take your stem cells even just down the hall because the stem cells' liquid lunch has a way of sloshing around as you walk. It is stressful for both the cells and the scientist doing the walking as well. Picture me walking with a book on my head trying not to let it fall (posture!) and that is kind of how we look when we carry our stem cells around the halls of research institutes. Hands tightly gripped on their dish, pulse elevated, and eyes darting up and down. Maybe we would be better off if we balanced the stem cells in their dishes on our heads? Maybe not.

No matter how careful we are, the stem cells taken for a walk in our research institutes have a way of running into trouble. If your dog runs away from home or from the park, you can usually find them and bring them home. At worst, you go around the neighborhood and put up "lost" posters. But if you slosh your stem cells' liquid chow and some stem cells along with it out of the dish, not only can you make a biohazardous mess, but you are also losing the stem cells forever. Imagine if you had to rapidly walk your expensive and beloved pet fish around the neighborhood in an aquarium filled to the very top with water and no lid. You might have the neighbor's cat following you hoping that you accidentally slosh the goldfish out onto the sidewalk for them to make a quick snack out of it.

When you take your dog on a walk it usually has a lot of fun and plays games. If stem cells get to have anything like fun in their cellular lives, perhaps it is when they are taken out of the incubator to be studied by a couple different types of scientific methods: being "centrifuged" and "being sorted". These two "games" are akin to a trip to the cellular amusement park.

When stem cells are centrifuged or "spun" as we call it in the lab, they are rotated around very fast until they sink to the bottom of a tube (due to their higher density than the media or saline solution that they are suspended in) so you can purify them.

I imagine the stem cells gradually spinning around faster and faster, much the same as kids on those spinning carnival rides. While the worst that might happen to a kid is that after the ride they are dizzy or barf, stem cells sometimes die after being spun even just a bit too fast or for an excessively long time. Therefore, centrifugation is an extreme cellular thrill ride to put it mildly. Imagine if planted by the spinning cups ride at the state fair that you are about to let your kid take a ride on there is a sign that says, "Warning: 1 in 20 children never return alive from this ride."

I guess it would not be a popular ride.

Perhaps more fun, even if just as risky for stem cells, is something called "sorting". Sorting is a method where you make stem cells glow in the dark and then the flow cytometer (aka "sorting machine") separates out the glowers from the non-glowers. This is a very technically useful way that we can purify stem cells as well as study their properties. The machine is called "flow cytometer" because the stem cells are made to flow in liquid and "cytometer" just means, "cell measurer".

The flow cytometer separates cells into different populations in a cool way. It accomplishes this first by sucking the stem cells, which are floating in a liquid, up into a tube inside the machine. Picture the character Augustus Gloop in *Charlie and Chocolate Factory* when he falls in the chocolate lake and gets sucked up into that tube. The stem cells swimming through a flow cytometer might feel like Augustus, although the diameter of the tubes in the cytometer are designed so that the cells, which lack the girth of Augustus, do not get stuck. After that the sorting machine shoots the cells inside a stream of liquid through a laser beam to make them glow before they plop down into various specific collection tubes depending on how they did or did not glow.

Talk about a wild ride!

Not only do they get to shine, but also I always imagine stem cells enjoying this wild ride, kind of like a cross between laser tag, a water slide, and finally Splash Mountain at Disneyland.

What determines which cells glow (and to what extent) and which do not inside the flow cytometer when it shoots them with the laser? To a large extent it depends on what experiment is going on, but the general approach is to take advantage of those membrane proteins that were discussed earlier. Researchers have antibodies that tightly bind to specific cell membrane proteins expressed only on stem cells for example. The cells are incubated with the antibodies prior to sorting so that trillions of antibodies bind specifically to the proteins on the surface of stem cells. The antibodies are special because they are fused to (we call it "conjugated") fancy glow-in-the-dark, fluorescent proteins that light up almost any color of rainbow you want when they are hit by laser light of a specific wavelength. Imagine a stem cell coated with a shag carpet of trillions of antibodies carrying green fluorescent protein shining bright green as a laser zaps it just enough to light it up, but not enough (we hope) to kill it. That stem cell then goes with the flow into a tube that you marked "stem cells". A neighboring cell floating in the stream of liquid that stays dark when hit by the laser may go into another tube or the trash.

Where is the stem cell going to sleep?

With pet dogs you at least in theory have choices about where they sleep. For example, you can let them say inside at night or they can have a doghouse. If they chew up your slippers you can give them the boot outside, not that I would ever do that to Elvis.

Stem cells not only must have the most expensive food, but they have the most discriminating taste when it comes to accommodations. Only expensive digs will do. They must live inside of a costly incubator, which must be located inside of a very expensive, well-maintained cellular "hotel" called a "tissue culture" room.

Often when we take stem cells out of their happy home to give them more of their media or to do experiments, we have to do it inside of a fancy piece of equipment called a "laminar flow hood", but we call it "the hood" for short in the lab. The hood keeps the stem cells' air and our air separate. In addition to our personal protective equipment of lab coat and such mentioned earlier, the hood protects stem cells from us, since we are crawling with nasty pathogens that would just love to multiple in their stem cell chow and kill them. But it also protects us from the stem cells because they too can harbor disease causing germs, particularly viruses.

Just as you do not want your dog wandering around in any old neighborhood, you need your stem cells to stay in the best hood. A good stem cell hood can be even more expensive than the incubators and takes up a lot of space, but when you are a fan of stem cells, you only want the best for them.

Inside the tissue culture room, whether inside the hood or inside the incubator, the final layer of protection is the plastic dish or a flask in which the stem cells live. The bottom of the dish is coated with a specific chemical that makes the stem cells happy to stick down (think cellular Velcro^{TM}) and grow as well as, in some cases, a feeder layer discussed earlier.

The stem cells are surrounded by their stem cell chow and grow together, usually in colonies. Stem cells like to grow in bunches in the lab most often because they trade proteins and other molecules that make each other happy. Very communal. Still the laboratory "dog house" for stem cells is no real niche. The physiochemical environment of stem cells in the lab is also profoundly different in many ways than the natural niche. For example, oxygen tension in a lab incubator is almost always hyperphysiological or too high because it is sourced simply from room air. Evidence suggests that room air levels of oxygen make stem cells grown in labs a bit unhealthy and less stem-like.

Over time, this excess of oxygen might tend to promote accumulation of mutations as well, due at least in part to high levels of free radicals. Within the endogenous stem cell niche, the level of oxygen is usually relatively low (only a few percent) as compared to ambient levels in the air. Interestingly stem cells prefer these low oxygen levels even if as a whole organism our lungs need the much higher ambient levels. For this reason, some stem cell labs have paid tens of thousands of dollars for specialized equipment to grow their stem cells in "low oxygen" conditions that are more niche-like.

Scientists also take measures to try to maintain a stable pH in the media of stem cells growing in our labs. To this end, we add chemicals called "buffers" to the cell media that make it somewhat resistant to fluctuations in pH. Further, we pipe in 5% carbon dioxide into the incubators, where it mixes with room air that filters in, because this also tends to stabilize pH at a near physiological 7.4 level.

Who will take care of the stem cell when we are on vacation?

Wait, stem cell scientists are not allowed to take vacations. Oh, shh, I was not supposed to reveal that secret. Actually scientists do now and then escape from the lab, leaving our poor stem cells behind. We experience some guilt about it. I feel that way when I go on a trip to a stem cell conference and have to leave Elvis at home.

In the lab world, we worry when we are gone on a trip because it is notorious for stem cells to die when their "owners" are gone. You head out of the lab and upon your return you find that your stem cells are dead or differentiated. Whoever was taking care of the cells for you invariably smiles a crooked smile, shrugs their shoulders, and moves on to their own lab experiments after giving you the bad news. They have probably experienced the same thing when they handed over care of their cells to someone else in the lab. Still, the vast majority of the time the stem cells are just fine when we return from trips even if the memories of the few times they did not fare so well are the ones that stick in our minds over the years.

How will you know if the stem cell is sick and what will you do about it?

Stem cells would make very sensitive pets, quite prone to chronic sickliness. As mentioned above, short trips can make them sick or be fatal. But even if you leave them alone and do everything right by them, it is still not unusual for them to get sick or to up and die on you for no apparent reason. When stem cells get sick, it is usually a bacterial, viral or fungal infection just like what might strike your dog or, in fact, you. But most often there is no remedy in the case of sick stem cells.

Imagine a big strong dog that does not want to go to the Vet (somehow they always know it is coming, don't they?) You are trying to pull it out the car door on a leash, straining against its collar. Our dog Elvis does that. She hates going to the vet and as a nearly 100 pound dog made mostly of muscle, she can put up great resistance. One time the Vet even had to give Elvis her treatment in the parking lot. Stem cells that get sick do not put up a fight, but they cannot be used for experiments so that is the end of the road for them.

There is another way that stem cells can get sick and that is they can spontaneously differentiate to transform themselves into non-stem cells. What a nasty trick, huh? Imagine your favorite pet poodle, which you have tenderly raised for years and that always sleeps at your bedside. You feed her the best food too. One morning you wake up and find that little Sugar during the night changed into a mutt or even worse an alligator that now is looking at you hungrily? Stem cells will not try to eat you, but it is just as painful for us scientists when the cells spontaneously transform into non-stem cells. All that hard work wasted. Of course, stem cell differentiation specifically when it is desired and controlled experimentally by scientists is a positive thing.

The only good news is that getting rid of these rebellious or sick stem cells is as easy as flushing your dead pet goldfish down the drain. Euthanasia comes in the form of a blast of bleach and then it is bye-bye. So for stem cells there is no Vet. At the first sign of trouble, they are history.

What are we going to name the stem cells?

Our dog Elvis had that unusual (given that she is a girl dog) name when we rescued her. It was given to her because she was born on the human Elvis' birthday.

Scientists love to name things with funny names too. This includes genes, proteins, and even cells.

Sometimes the name has some secret meaning, such as referring to the researchers themselves or their kid by their initials or a nickname. Fruit fly researchers are particularly notorious for picking the most outlandish names for things they discover, such as naming a growth factor "Sonic HedgeHog" after the cartoon character, but the stem cell field has its own naming issues and the most problematic is the reliance on acronyms.

Most stem cells of a specific type are named "X Stem Cells", where the X is supposed to tell you what they are all about, so they often end up with the acronym "XSC". Some examples include MSC (mesenchymal stem cell) and neural stem cells, aka "NSC". The name "iPS cells" was a bit refreshing since it did not end in SC, but now scientists are often calling them "iPSC" instead of "iPS cells".

What exactly will we get out of having these stem cells?

What will a lab get out of taking care of and studying specific stem cells? This can be a million-dollar question.

For dogs it is kind of more obvious. Dogs are "man's best friend". They will come when you call. They will sit and maybe even shake hands. If you are really lucky they will roll over upon command. They can also protect you. More than anything pet dogs such as our Elvis are like members of the family. Service dogs can even make patients feel better in ways that doctors and researchers can measure.

Stem cells do have some pretty amazing tricks of their own though that put the most well behaved spaniel at a dog show to shame. If you simply spike their stem cell chow with Vitamin A for example, you can get them to turn into neurons! That is a pretty neat trick. It would akin to adding some pureed magic carrots to your dog's chow and the next day your Chihuahua has transformed into a Wooly Mammoth. This stem cell pet trick (I am referring to "differentiation") is really that mind-boggling of a change. Depending on what supplement you add to the pluripotent stem cell chow, you can generate an almost limitless number of cell types if you are working with pluripotent stem cells. In the case of the transformation of stem cells into neurons, if you grow enough of them and for long enough they will form a neural network or array, complete with active synapses and dendrites. This is akin to growing a micro brain in a dish!

This "differentiation" pluripotent stem cell pet trick means that in theory you can use stem cells to make any cell type for fixing any diseased or injured organ if you could transplant the stem cells or their differentiated progeny into the damaged organ. Of course differentiation needs to be carefully induced and controlled, as scientists do not want stem cells spontaneously differentiating of their own accord into a haphazard collection of various cell types that are clinically and experimentally useless. As mentioned earlier, spontaneous uncontrolled differentiation of stem cells is a recipe for an experimental dead end.

In terms of more pet-like tricks, stem cells are really good at sitting and staying. If I go into our tissue culture room and say "sit" or "stay" to our stem cells, they do not move a muscle, unless they have been differentiated into beating cardiac muscle, which is a beautiful thing to see![i] But staying is about the only pet-like trick stem cells can do and in fact at a microscopic level the stem cells still crawl around.

Ultimately, however, stem cells may give something quite valuable and very serious to society: new treatments and cures for major diseases and injuries. Think rescue dogs like St. Bernards, service dogs, and Lassie all rolled into one. Stem cells would make difficult, high maintenance pets, but how many pets have the promise to one day cure humanity of so many tragic diseases through a revolution in medicine?

What Could Go Wrong in the Lab?

Despite our best efforts to make stem cells happy in the lab, there are compelling reasons to believe that cells grown in labs outside of the body may change in substantial and clinically meaningful ways. I outline in detail eight simple reasons why one should not get an experimental, unlicensed procedure based on laboratory grown stem cells outside of a clinical trial in Chapter 9.

During amplification in culture, the healthy heterogeneity (degree of variability in a population) of endogenous natural stem cell cultures often changes and becomes limited by what is called "clonal expansion" of certain "super" cells that outcompete others. Clonal expansion means that over time in a diverse population, one cell type may eventually take over the population because it has traits that allow it to outcompete the other cells. Think of it as cellular evolution in action, but "survival of the fittest" within cell populations does not always give us lab-grown cell populations that scientists, doctors, and patients would prefer.

---

[i]http://www.youtube.com/watch?v=4R-q3r03LkA

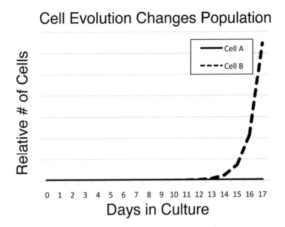

Figure 5.3. Example of how in a culture, one cell type can take over the culture in a period as short as about two weeks. If the stem cell culture has two main cell types (A and B) we will assume that one, in this case cell type B, grows moderately faster (50%).

In a hypothetical example of problems associated with clonal expansion, let us consider the case of a stem cell culture that at the start has two main types of cells: A and B. In this scenario, A and B are generally the same type of stem cell, but B cells grow 50% faster than A on average. Normal stem cells on average divide to become two cells about once a day, a process we call "population doubling". After only 10 population doublings in our hypothetical culture, based on their different rates of doubling, type B cells will be 58-fold overrepresented in culture relative to type A cells. After only 7 more doublings, type B cell overrepresentation approaches 1,000-fold (see Figure 5.3) and basically the culture is entirely made up of type B cells.

This hypothetical example serves to illustrate how rapid cell evolution can occur during in vitro expansion of stem cells in the lab. This process also favors cells that resist differentiation and apoptosis (cell death), events that when they occur end a given cell's contribution to the final cellular population. Therefore, after even a relatively short period of just a few weeks in culture, an amplified stem cell population will contain an overrepresentation of cells that tend to have a certain cellular personality: they grow more rapidly, resist apoptosis, and are less prone to differentiate than their original endogenous cellular neighbors.

Unfortunately, all three of these cellular attributes would tend to make cells behave in a manner more analogous to cancer cells.

In other words, the longer that scientists and doctors grow stem cells in the lab, the higher the probability that the population at the end (often to be transplanted into patients) will behave more like cancer cells. In my opinion, this reality is one crucial justification for the regulation of laboratory-grown stem cells as a drug and for mandating safety testing prior to their clinical use (discussed further in Chapter 7).

Another concern about in vitro laboratory expansion of cells is the potential contamination of cells during the time they spend in the laboratory. Stem cells may be contaminated in a number of ways in the lab. The warm, nutrient rich environment in which we grow stem cells in the lab is ideal for the growth of opportunistic pathogens including bacteria, viruses, and fungi. While there are laboratory tests that can be used to monitor stem cell transplants for pathogen contamination, absent FDA regulatory oversight, it remains unclear if non-compliant stem cell clinics follow strict standard operating procedures (SOPs) to minimize the risks of such infections and monitor for them. Note that sometimes pathogen infections of stem cells are obvious during growth in the lab, while at other times they are subtle and might only manifest explosively once the cells are transplanted into patients.

Any tissue culture facility in which cells are grown from multiple individual patients (common in the non-compliant, for-profit stem cell clinic world) and by multiple operators, runs a risk of viral infection of their cultures that could raise safety concerns. A pertinent example is the recent case of the XMRV retrovirus, which was erroneously linked to prostate cancer in a report [1]. Subsequently it was shown [2, 3] that the apparent presence of XMRV was an artifact of laboratory contamination. If clinical laboratory technicians are not careful, one person's cells can also easily become contaminated with another person's cells if they are both grown in the same lab as well with potentially disastrous consequences after transplantation.

Cells grown in culture also are frequently exposed to xenobiotic (foreign, non-human) antigens in the laboratory as discussed earlier. This contamination can occur when cells are grown in fetal bovine serum (FBS). While the FDA does allow some use of FBS in the culturing of cells intended for clinical trial use, permission must be obtained a priori from the FDA in the context of pre-clinical and early phase clinical trials. Some point-of-care, for-profit stem cell clinics use FBS to expand their stem cell products without FDA permission.

What this all means is that in an average day in the life of a laboratory stem cell, it is far more likely to change its personality and to be become contaminated in potentially dangerous ways. In contrast, its endogenous stem cell counterpart that is safely tucked away in the niche inside the body remains protected.

The Black Sheep of the Family: Cancer Stem Cells

There is another kind of stem cell in the "family" (see family portrait again in Figure 5.1). It is the black sheep of the family: the cancer stem cell. As mentioned in Chapter 1, when stem cells are damaged or mutated they usually die, but sometimes can turn into cancer stem cells, a type of stem cell that has the frightening power to develop an entire tumor from a single cell.

How might this happen?

The external and even internal forces threatening our endogenous stem cells are formidable. The dangers to the health of our stem cells include radiation, chemicals in our environment, and even toxic substances that our own bodies and cells create. These factors can damage or kill any cell including stem cells. One result of the damage to our stem cells is an acceleration of the rate at which our stem cell numbers decrease via cell death over the time we live. Unfortunately this process not only contributes to aging via cell death, but can also lead to cancer when these elements damage stem cells without actually killing them.

Most often when our endogenous stem cells are damaged they very conveniently self-destruct (also known as undergoing apoptosis or programmed cell death) or are eliminated by the built-in safety net of our immune system because they are recognized as unhealthy. But occasionally an altered stem cell somehow can survive in a damaged form. Every so often one of these damaged survivors turns into a cancer stem cell.

Even though cancer stem cells are "self" in the sense that they are almost entirely identical to their normal cellular kin, their instability and the changes that they do possess (e.g. mistakenly a nuclear protein can be expressed as a cell membrane antigen) lead them to attract the attention of the immune system and they end up being killed. But not always. Some escape from immune cells in a disappearing act that would make legendary escape artist Houdini proud.

After evading both self-destruction and being killed by our immune systems, every so often these damaged stem cells turns to the "dark side". Much the same as Anakin Skywalker in the *Star Wars* saga takes on the new name "Darth Vader" after nearly being killed and turning to the dark side, normal stem cells can become so-called cancer stem cells after being injured. Cancer stem cells are the most dangerous cells known to humanity. A single cancer stem cell possesses the power to create an entire new tumor that may contain hundreds of billions of cells, all derived from that one cancer stem cell.

Cancer stem cells are also thought to be a prime cause of therapeutic resistance to cancer treatments and as a result, a main reason for cancer recurrence. Cancer stem cells are stealthy and can go into what is termed a "quiescent" state in which the cell is in essence asleep. Such sleeper cells are particularly resistant to what doctors use to treat cancer patients such as chemo and radiation, which largely target and kill actively proliferating cells.

This hibernation also helps the cancer stem cells evade the immune system. As a result, a high priority in both stem cell and cancer research today is the development of new methods to identify cancer stem cells and specifically kill them. On an average day in the life of a cancer stem cell it may seem outwardly to be a very benign "quiet" cell, but when it becomes active, watch out!

Amongst the features of a typical day in the life of a cancer stem cell there are some clues as to why it is so dangerous. Cancer stem cells can still be dependent upon a stem cell niche, but it is thought that this dependency is far less absolute. What this means is that, cancer stem cells can survive and retain their corrupted stem-like properties in less than ideal niches that may not have all the characteristics required of an endogenous stem cell niche to promote normal stem cell survival.

Cancer stem cells may also be able to persist entirely outside of a niche for days, weeks, or even years at a time. This transient period of time "niche-less" could be in the blood stream or elsewhere before the cancer stem cell moves on some place else. An endogenous stem cell or even a laboratory-produced stem cell is far less likely to survive this period outside the niche. What this means is that in the average day for a cancer stem cell, it may be less likely to be found in a proper niche. This flexibility in terms of tolerance of different locations makes cancer stem cells far more likely to cause cancer metastasis.

Cancer stem cells are also more migratory than the average stem cell as well as than the average cancer cell. Therefore, even over a period of time as short as one day a cancer stem cell may be in more than one place. The migratory nature of cancer stem cells also increases their threat to our health because of metastasis.

The addiction of endogenous and laboratory stem cells to growth factors is something that cancer stem cells frequently have beaten as well with potentially disastrous consequences. Cancer stem cells are far more likely to survive in an environment with lower growth factor levels that may occur in various locations in the body. One mechanism by which cancer stem cells escape this addiction is by having abnormal growth factor receptors on their cell membrane surface that are locked into the "on" mode even in the absence of growth factors.

Overall, the average day in the life a cancer stem cell is less predictable than the other types of stem cells. The fact that cancer stem cells are less dependent on the niche and growth factors gives them the independence to cause trouble.

Summary

The average days in the lives of the three stem cells discussed in this chapter give you a sense of what can go right and what can go wrong with stem cells. The environment in which the cell finds itself has a dramatic influence on whether it behaves well or badly in the sense of having functional properties that are clinically desirable. Overall, a general rule of thumb is that the less time that a cell spends outside the niche or outside the body in a laboratory, the more akin to a healthy, normal stem cell it is likely to be. But for a number of possible stem cell medical applications, some time in the lab is unavoidable.

References

1. Schlaberg, R, et al. (2009) XMRV is present in malignant prostatic epithelium and is associated with prostate cancer, especially high-grade tumors. *Proceedings of the National Academy of Sciences of the United States of America.* **106**:38:16351-6.
2. Lee, D, et al. (2012) In-Depth Investigation of Archival and Prospectively Collected Samples Reveals No Evidence for XMRV Infection in Prostate Cancer. *PLoS One.* 7:9:e44954.
3. Mendoza, R, et al. (2012) No biological evidence of XMRV in blood or prostatic fluid from prostate cancer patients. *PLoS One.* **7**:5:e36073.

Chapter 6

Aging: The Stem Cell Connection

Could stem cells stop or even reverse aging?

We all are born, get old, and die.

Human beings generally have been asking themselves the same universal questions about aging and death for thousands of years.

Why do we have to age?

What happens when we age?

Can we do anything about it?

Could we even perhaps escape death?

Much the same as the weather, throughout human history, aging has been something that people could just wonder or complain about, but there did not seem to be anything that they could do to substantially impact it even if they had the awareness and conscious desire to do so.

People would fantasize about ways to stop or reverse aging such as the mythical *Fountain of Youth* pursued by Spanish explorer Ponce de Leon and many others across the world, but the stark reality was that aging and ultimately death seemed mysterious, arbitrary, and unstoppable.

Remarkably that reality of being human that has spanned millennia is changing and a big part of this cosmic shift is spurred by stem cells.

Unlike the billions of humans that have come before us, in the coming decades we will be in a unique position related to aging. Now instead of just complaining about aging, in coming decades we might be able to actually do something about it and stem cells hold the key. Through a better understanding of the aging process and the role of stem cells we may all be able to live longer, healthier lives.

But we cannot get ahead of ourselves.

For example, the stem cell anti-aging clinics out there in the world today cannot achieve what they claim in the way of slowing or even reversing aging via stem cell transplants. That is pure hype and snake oil at this point. Yet that does not stop them from collecting large sums of money from patients around the world.

The other day a lady stopped me in the elevator and said, "Hey, you are that stem cell guy, right?" She continued, "Stem cells are big in the Philippines. We get twelve IV injections of sheep stem cells and suddenly we are younger. We look younger and feel younger. Keep up the good work!"

I did not have the time to tell her that what she had described for me was completely bogus and even quite dangerous. I have received phone calls and emails that largely expressed the same message as the elevator lady.

Most stem cell anti-aging clinics in the US do IV transplantation of stem cells, but usually human cells, not sheep or goat or pig cells. But I have heard of each of the three farmyard varieties being commonly used by dubious clinics in various countries. There is no scientific or even basic common sense reason why injecting a bunch of stem cells (whether human or otherwise) into the blood stream will make you younger or stop aging, but millions are being spent on such therapies. I strongly recommend against them.

It turns out that as much as treatments using stem cells of other species sounds like snake oil, using other people's stem cells may be even more dangerous given the risk of transmission of human-specific diseases such as Hepatitis or cancer if you are immunosuppressed. This is not to say that injections of stem cells from barnyard animals into human patients are something that I advocate as safe. I do not.

Despite all this quackery, there are legitimate research efforts ongoing to better understand the links between stem cells and aging. In addition, stem cell technology may someday in principle help us truly fight aging. That day is not today or even sometime next year, but eventually that day will come in a time span measured most likely in decades.

Still, much sooner than that, a greater understanding of stem cells could allow for battling aging in real ways for the first time in history.

In theory transplants of organs produced in the lab via stem cells could delay aging or death as well. We are not there yet in terms of organ replacement via stem cell-produced fully-grown organs or supplementation of the functions of deteriorating old, injured, or diseased organs with new, healthy mini-organs. However, these ideas seem plausible in the coming decades (discussed in more depth in Chapter 13).

Scientists are taking the possibility of stem cell-based organ growth seriously and so should you. Another very real possibility that could be realized in a decade or less is the development of anti-aging drugs that target endogenous stem cells to keep them healthier and more abundant.

As technology advances, we may reevaluate aging and think about it in new ways. I believe there is already evidence to support such innovative thinking and here I propose *The Stem Cell Theory of Aging*. To be clear, it is just a theory, but there are some data to support it and I believe it helps us think about aging in a whole new, helpful way.

According to this theory, our aging is directly proportional to how many stem cells we have and their relative degree of healthiness. *The Stem Cell Theory of Aging* tells us that if we do all we can to maintain a robust population of healthy stem cells, we at least have a better chance of aging more slowly and leading a healthier life. I admit this is speculative, but it is a thought-provoking notion. As our stem cells metaphorically slip down through the hourglass over time in this model, we age proportionately (Figure 6.1).

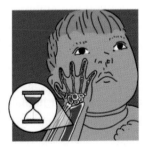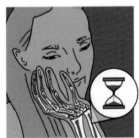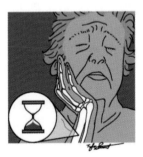

Figure 6.1. The Stem Cell Theory of Aging. Instead of grains of sand going through the hourglass, the purple objects are stem cells. As they run through the hourglass we age. When they run out, we die. Illustration by Taylor Seamount.

The basic idea of the stem cell aging theory is that aging does not just correlate with human beings having fewer stem cells, but also that aging is in part actually *caused* by the reduction in healthy stem cell populations. The notion that as our stem cells age we may also in parallel age as an organism is not entirely new. For example, there was a recent article in the journal *Cell Stem Cell* exploring the possible connections between stem cells and aging [1]. In a sense, I am going out on a limb in this chapter arguing that there is indeed a strong connection between stem cells and aging.

To explain the full logic behind this notion, we have to start at the beginning of human development and discuss the different roles of the stem cells that we have throughout a typical human lifespan. Few of us think about it, but we all start our existence as a single stem cell: the fertilized egg. This remarkable stem cell, the one cell embryo, is more powerful than any other known type of cell. It is *totipotent*, meaning it can form every possible type of human cell. In the stem cell field, "potent" refers to how many other kinds of cells a stem cell can make and "toti" means "everything". This one totipotent stem is responsible for producing the trillions of cells of the human body during development.

However, it is not infallible or somehow magical. In fact, often times this fertilized egg or even the early multi-celled embryo that it turns into over the course of the first few days of a pregnancy fails to thrive and no human being is created.

The rate at which these early embryos fail for one reason or another is thought to be quite high with half-to-two-thirds of early human embryos failing.[i] Many of these embryos simply dissolve without the woman even knowing she was pregnant, whereas other times this embryo failure explains a woman's late period that does not go on to pregnancy.

If we focus on what happens when things do go right, the process is quite remarkable. The first thing that occurs after fertilization in human development is that the zygote, undergoes cell division, turning into two

---

[i]http://www.whattoexpect.com/pregnancy/pregnancy-health/complications/miscarriage.aspx

new identical "daughter" cells. Each of these two cells then divides turning collectively into four cells, and so on.

At the eight-cell embryonic stage, each of those eight stem cells is identical and all are able to form a whole embryo. Prior to this point during the earliest days of human pregnancy, the embryo's cells act like copy machines churning out new "cloned" versions of themselves. At the eight-cell stage, if one of those cells happens to accidentally separate from the other seven without causing all the cells and in turn the pregnancy to fail, the result is identical twins: one produced from the clump of seven cells and the other from the one cell that strayed. Identical twins are the only known example of human cloning, in this case natural. The prospect of laboratory-based human reproductive cloning will be discussed later in Chapter 12.

Getting back to our hypothetical natural pregnancy, a major change happens after the eight-cell stage. As the process goes from sixteen to thirty-two cells and so on, some cells start behaving differently. All the cells present are still stem cells, but some are already committed to defined fates. Some of these cells lose pluripotency and are already on their way to specific differentiated fates.

In humans at the hundred-cell stage, known as the blastocyst embryo, about half of the cells are destined to form the embryo proper and if things go right, ultimately an entire adult human body (for actual images of these early human embryos see Figure 2.3 in Chapter 2). The other cells will become extraembryonic tissues such as the placenta. This is the stage from which embryonic stem cells are made from leftover laboratory-produced blastocysts from in vitro fertilization (IVF) procedures.

Focusing in vivo, as the stem cells of the embryo continue to divide and diverge in terms of their ultimate pathways or fates, their numbers increase at a rapid clip, roughly doubling once or twice a day. Despite this divergence in cellular identity, essentially all the cells of the early embryo are still stem cells, just of more and more diverse kinds with different potencies.

At some point about halfway through in utero development, at what is called *mid-gestation*, the relative number of stem cells we have starts a downward trend. More and more cells become devoted to specialized functions and entirely lose stem-like properties. By the time we are born and take our first breaths, the vast majority of the cells in our bodies are not stem cells anymore, but this is entirely normal and is by nature's design. We need those specialized, non-stem cells that make up our organs such as our hearts and brains, for example.

The primary job of stem cells is as body builders, in a literal sense that is, since their first task is to construct our bodies. When we are born, that bodybuilding is mostly completed. We have grown billions of times in mass going from a single cell to become a living, breathing, thinking human being with trillions of cells.

While of course we still have more growing to do from a newborn baby through the end of adolescence when most of us stop growing, the relative postnatal change in human mass — just 20-30 fold — is more modest compared to what has happened in utero. We also still have billions of stem cells at birth, but proportionately our non-stem cells as babies greatly outnumber our stem cells, whereas earlier in development the embryo was entirely or almost entirely stem cells.

Throughout our childhood we retain a significant population of stem cells. At some point within a decade of the onset of puberty, our growth rapidly slows and eventually stops. We no longer get taller. If we get heavier, it is mostly due to accumulation of fat. Our body is built. This does not mean that our body is static as many changes are still ongoing such as our brain maturing, but the first job of our stem cells is essentially completely done. They have grown each of us into a mature body, a truly astonishing accomplishment for our stem cells.

At this point, the second stem cell job — maintaining us in a healthy, relatively youthful form — takes over. To achieve this goal, stem cells replace or repair our tissues as cells are lost and also replace their own populations too. Stem cells are especially vital for replacing cells that naturally die at a relatively rapid pace such as skin, gut, and blood cells. These cells are also notable as being the ones most sensitive to radiation or toxin damage precisely because the cells in these tissues are normally rapidly lost and must be replaced quickly in a stem cell-dependent process. This is why radiation or chemotherapy treatments for certain forms of cancer have the most pronounced side effects in the skin (hair falls out), gut (various symptoms including diarrhea), and blood system (e.g. anemia, bruising, and bleeding).

During adult life, stem cells produce new differentiated cells that replace cells that have lived their designated life spans or that are damaged (with mutations) or sick (e.g. virus-infected). Cell replacement via our own endogenous stem cells maintains our tissues in a state of homeostasis for decades after our late teens. As adults we do not need to grow taller or have our organs get bigger so stem cells coordinate a precise homeostatic state. If we lose a billion cells from our skin in one day, remarkably stem cells orchestrate the production of exactly one billion replacements. When we lose a trillion blood cells over the course of a few days that is how many new ones are made. Not any more or any less, which in either case could cause disease.

How stem cells "know", in other words how they are programmed at a molecular level, to function so meticulously remains a subject of intense investigation in research labs around the world. Part of the reason for the great interest in precisely figuring out how homeostatic stem cell activity is controlled is because if we understand that process then in theory we can make drugs that will turn stem cells on or off. Such drugs could be quite powerful ways to not only treat patients via targeting endogenous stem cells, but also to modulate the activity of laboratory-grown stem cells prior to transplant.

When this endogenous stem cell homeostatic system goes awry, producing more or less cells than are needed, it leads to illness. For example in the skin too many cells can lead to psoriasis or in a more extreme example, skin cancer. Too few cells may cause aging of the skin or failure of skin to maintain a barrier to the outside environment.

Stem cells also heal tissues that are injured or diseased. If we get sick, stem cells ramp up our immune systems, creating trillions of new infection-fighting blood cells to defend us against pathogens such as bacteria and viruses.

This second job of stem cells, essentially fulfilling the maintenance contract of human bodies, goes on the rest of our lives, but with varying degrees of success.

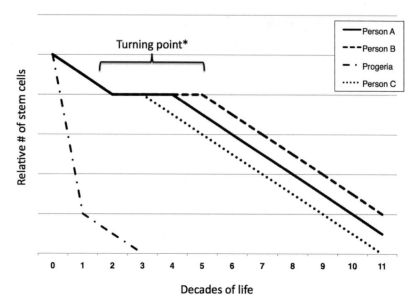

Figure 6.2. Hypothetical graph of the stem cell turning point as part of The Stem Cell Theory of Aging. Person A is an average human who reaches the turning point somewhere in a window between thirties and early forties. Person B is a hypothetical individual who either because of lifestyle or genetics or both, has a later stem cell turning point, retains more stem cells longer, and lives longer on average. Person C is a being who either because of lifestyle or genetics or both, has an earlier stem cell turning point, retains fewer stem cells, and lives shorter on average. These hypothetical people are compared to a Progeria patient who either does not have a stem cell turning point at all or it occurs transiently at a very young age. *The Stem Cell Turning point is defined as the time during mature adult life when our number of stem cells starts to steadily decline leading us to age.

While fulfilling this role, stem cells themselves get damaged, worn out, and die as they fix and protect us. As a result, while they are still healthy they must every so often make more stem cells, creating their own replacements. They are naturally programmed to do this, a process called "self-renewal", on a regular basis. They do it amazingly well such that the number of stem cells in our bodies remains relatively constant for a couple decades after we stop growing.

However, the stem cell aging theory predicts that at some point in our adult lives, somewhere in our thirties to forties, we reach an unfortunate turning point. I call this *the stem cell turning point* (Figure 6.2), and I believe it is the chief health-related turning point of our lives. One day, without even knowing it, the number of stem cells in our bodies no longer stays roughly steady at the healthy adult level. Instead, this number starts to consistently decline as the self-renewal process whereby more stem cells are made as replacements for old stem cells, starts to falter.

We are no longer quite as good at replacing our old stem cells and the numbers start slipping. This happens very slowly at first, but picks up pace as we age and continues until the day we die. There is a wealth of scientific evidence that stem cell numbers decline with age in many different tissues: blood [2], skin [3], muscle [4], and brain [5]. I do not believe this is a coincidence. Rather, the decrease in stem cells in organs with aging causes those organs to biologically age.

For some of us, the fateful day that we die will come earlier as the result of some acute event such as a car accident or heart attack. For others, we will die of "old age". However, I believe that the process of aging before death is directly correlated with and caused by our declining numbers of healthy stem cells.

In a way, of course we age every day of our lives even as children since each day that we are alive, potentially our cells can be damaged or acquire mutations, but up until the day when we cross the stem cell turning point, most of us remain generally youthful and healthy. The "aging" that we do prior to that turning point is just a normal part of being a living, relatively youthful human being. But once we pass the stem cell turning point, we really start to age in the sense of declining health.

During the period of our lives after the stem cell turning point, there are fewer stem cells in our organs and those remaining stem cells have more trouble with their job of tissue maintenance. For example, after the turning point when our skin gets exposed to UV radiation from sunlight or gets scratched or bruised, it may no longer bounce back the way it used it. Also, as we naturally shed skin each day, the new skin that replaces it is not so youthful. As we lose blood cells, our hematopoietic stem cells are no longer quite as good at replacing them. When we get sick, our immune system does not ramp up as robustly as it used to so we are not only more likely to get sick in the first place, but also we tend to stay sick longer.

After the stem cell turning point, hair stem cells, which are responsible for replacing our hair when it falls out, do not do as effective a job so we gradually lose hair.

The stem cells whose job it is to make hair pigment become depleted in numbers too after the stem cell turning point so the real underlying color of our hair strands (which consist of simply white or slightly yellowish proteins when not containing extra pigments) starts showing up. Hair begins to look gray.

The stem cells in our muscles that normally fix them or that help "pump us up" literally growing more muscle when we exercise, become fewer. As a result, the percentage of our body that is muscle goes down and when we pull a muscle it does not heal as well.

Most of the changes that together constitute what we call "aging" may be linked to fewer or less functional stem cells.

The Stem Cell Theory of Aging that I am proposing here argues that the later that that turning point occurs and the slower that the decline of our stem cells proceeds afterwards, the slower we should age. The logical question is then, "How do we either delay the stem cell turning point, or if we have already passed it, how do we in essence push back the clock and slow aging?"

There is no one "right" answer to this question and a great deal depends on what is discovered from current and future research on stem cells and aging. Also, the answer may be that we cannot push back the clock at all via stem cell-based interventions. However, I am hopeful that in coming decades we will figure out ways to slow aging via stem cell technology. We also need to be more aware of the role of stem cells in our health and aging. If understand the aging process more fully then we become better equipped to find ways to delay aging. As the expression goes "know your enemy".

One stem cell-based approach to tackling aging that I strongly support is deceptively simple: work to take better care of our resident populations of all of our cells including our stem cells through lifestyle changes such as healthier diets and exercise. In fact, exercise has been shown to increase stem cell numbers in the brain [6] and other organs [7].

A second, more controversial idea is that stem cell transplants may some day slow aging. As enticing as this second idea may be to some, to date there is no scientific evidence that it actually works. I absolutely do not believe that it is effective in its current form and it could be dangerous.

What does my stem cell aging theory share with and how is it different from other theories about aging?

Many other theories of aging have been proposed over the years, and one thing they all share is the defeatist mentality that aging is unavoidable. The simplest and most popular theory is that our bodies wear out much the same as machines that can only be used a certain number of times. There is some truth to this theory, but notably unlike a machine, our bodies have the capacity to repair themselves through stem cells.

Imagine if after a fender bender, your car repaired itself such that the next morning when you went into the garage all the dents were gone and the broken headlight had been replaced with a new one that your car had grown itself? What our body does to maintain itself is no less miraculous, but we generally take it for granted. Our ability to heal ourselves, keeping ourselves from wearing out, is very dependent on stem cells.

Another theory is that our cells have a built in molecular clock determined by genetics. In this way of thinking, stem cells can only live so long and that length is determined by the speed with which the molecular clock runs. We see evidence of this in normal cells that we grow in the lab, which barring immortalization will only divide a finite number of times before permanently stopping.

One potential cellular and molecular aging clock of sorts consists of special segments of DNA at the end of our chromosomes called *telomeres*. Telomeres protect our DNA from damage. As we age telomeres tend to get shorter and shorter. If they get too short, the DNA becomes damaged and the cell dies. An enzyme called telomerase counteracts telomere shortening. Telomere shortening has been proposed as an aging timer of sorts. But mice that have no telomerase enzyme and have shorter telomeres live a normal lifespan, arguing against the telomere clock theory being absolute [8]. Nonetheless it is clear that telomeres protect our DNA and since they do tend to get shorter as we age, I believe there is a connection to aging, but as with many elements of biology, there are likely redundant mechanisms at work. There may also be other types of molecular or cellular clocks in our bodies that affect aging.

Regardless of the cause of aging, we all in effect carry two "ages" around with us.

First, there is our chronological age meaning the actual number of years that we have been alive. This is a number we cannot control of course. We all also have a second age that is one that we can perhaps change to some degree at least: our biological age. Our biological age is the relative condition of our bodies compared to the average of all human beings. For example, in the case of patients with the Progeria rapid aging syndromes, a "child" of ten years of chronological age, might have a biological age of 70 years because his body has aged in fast forward.

Progeria makes people age kind of akin to dogs in fast forward. This means that despite the fact that he has only lived ten years, the body of our hypothetical child suffering from Progeria has aged seven times faster than normal. As a result, the physiological condition of his organs and his cells is very similar to that of a seventy-year old man. Even though his chronological age is ten, his biological age is seventy, highlighting that our biological age is far more relevant to our health and lifespan than our chronological age. He may have had a very early stem cell turning point or none at all (Figure 6.2).

Another example would be a hypothetical man with a chronological age of seventy, but who has taken remarkably good care of himself and perhaps was blessed with good genetic luck to keep relatively large populations of healthy stem cells even as he aged. As a result his biological age is closer to fifty and he has aged far more slowly than the average man. He likely went through the stem cell turning point later in life than most people, and ever since that time, perhaps the decline in his stem cells has been relatively slow. What this means is that his own decline, meaning aging, has been slower as well. We all know people who seem far older or far younger than their chronological age, and research suggests that people who appear younger actually live longer than those of the same age who look older.[ii]

[ii]http://news.bbc.co.uk/2/hi/health/8411329.stm

Unfortunately, Progeria syndromes are genetic conditions, meaning they are caused by mutations. They either spontaneously occur in utero or are inherited from parents, meaning that they may be impossible to entirely prevent. At this time, Progeria is largely not only incurable, but also untreatable. However, physicians and the families of patients with Progeria may help them live a relatively longer, healthier life by focusing on dietary and lifestyle changes that would help take care of their stem cells. Even though there is relatively little for medicine to offer Progeria patients, the molecular events that occur in these people can teach us a great deal about aging.

The mutations that result in premature aging syndromes often affect what goes on in the nuclei of our cells and in that way the integrity of our genomic DNA. In the most common form of Progeria, the disorder that is sometimes actually simply called "Progeria Syndrome" or "Hutchinson–Gilford Syndrome", patients have a mutation in a gene called *Laminin A* or LMNA [9]. The LMNA gene makes (or as we call it in biology "encodes") a protein of the same name whose job is to make an integral structural part of our cells' nuclear lamina or nuclear membrane. The function of the nuclear lamina is to protect our cells' nuclei and the DNA they each contain, the same kind of way that the cell membrane that we talked so much about in Chapter 5 protects the whole cell or that our skin protects our entire body from the outside world.

The mutation in LMNA that causes Progeria is remarkably small, changing only one amino acid in the entire protein. Amino acids are the building blocks of proteins, kind of like Legos™, and LMNA has 572 of them. Although the DNA mutation in Progeria results in the change of just 1 out of LMNA's 572 amino acids, the end result is that the mutant LMNA protein is rendered unusable by our cells. In turn the nuclear membrane in Progeria patients as a whole cannot do its job of protecting our DNA.

Every time our cells divide, they must disassemble their nuclear lamina as they duplicate and segregate their DNA into two new daughter cells, which ultimately form new nuclear lamina of their own. It is thought that in some Progeria patients, the presence of the mutated LMNA protein interferes with this process. The end result is either cell death or if cells survive they have a dramatically higher rate of damaged

DNA. Because at any given time in our bodies, stem cells and their daughter progenitor cells are the most common type of dividing cell, one theory is that the LMNA mutation causes rapid aging by damaging and killing stem and progenitor cells. Cells that survive have a dramatically increased probability of acquiring additional mutations besides LMNA as well.

Most other Progeria Syndromes, including Werner's Syndrome, are also caused by mutations that in one way or another affect DNA integrity in cells including stem cells. Werner's Syndrome is the result of mutation of a gene called WRN, which encodes a protein of the same name that is a type of very cool, powerful enzyme called a "DNA helicase". In the cell nucleus, DNA helicases have a number of jobs, but most significantly they untangle and fix damaged DNA. DNA helicases are amazing proteins that act akin to spiders gliding around fixing the silken strands of their webs after say a bumblebee has crashed through them. DNA helicases ride around on DNA strands untangling and repairing the DNA strands. Radiation and chemicals such as reactive oxygen species crash into our DNA in a manner similar to that bee that damages the spider's web. Without properly functioning DNA helicases such as in Werner's Syndrome Patients [10], DNA rapidly accumulates mutations and this may translate into aging.

A key concept I take from research into Progeria syndromes is that mutated DNA in stem cells (and hence in all our cells since they all derive from stem cells and inherit their DNA from them) is not only a hallmark of aging, but also a primary cause of aging. Conversely, keeping your stem cell DNA undamaged is likely to fight aging. Whether human beings can willfully do something to protect their DNA via their lifestyles is hotly debated. But our body has an arsenal of defenders that automatically protect our DNA such as LMNA and also a team of molecular medics including the DNA helicases that fix damage when it occurs. We also have natural antioxidants such as Vitamin D produced in our skin that protect DNA.

Progeria has much to teach us and paradoxically, it also proves an important, even encouraging concept: the aging process is not fixed in stone either way.

We do not have to age at a certain, unchangeable rate. For the vast majority of us, heredity is not destiny when it comes to aging. Genetic diseases such as those that cause Progeria can accelerate aging, but how we live our lives can in principle at least slow it down somewhat too. Although genetics plays an undeniably influential role in aging and health, even identical twins do not age in exactly the same manner. How we live our lives and especially how we treat our stem cells, directly influence our speed of aging. I believe that "antigeria", slowing or fighting aging, is realistic, if we take better care of our cellular health. Over the course of the next decade or two, I think that stem cell research will teach us how to do this and drugs may be discovered that slow stem cell aging and in turn human aging.

But caution is in order.

As mentioned above, today there are clinics in the US and around the world offering stem cell-based, experimental anti-aging procedures. If you are willing and able to pay the price tags (typically thousands of dollars) at these clinics, they will give you stem cell therapies that they claim will slow or even reverse the aging process, but sadly these therapies will not help you and could do the ultimate in speed aging.

Kill you.

Stem Cell Banking: Another Way to Battle Aging?

Another model invoking stem cells and aging that many people are literally banking on anticipates a smarter or sicker future. Based on the notions that future technology will have better ways to use stem cells and that younger stem cells are better, some people today freeze away their stem cells in biological banks for potential future use when they are sick.

Stem cell banking means using cryogenic technology to deposit and in theory indefinitely store stem cells for some anticipated future use. When I was a kid I remember hearing about people having themselves frozen or even just their heads frozen shortly after death. The idea was to cheat mortality by preserving oneself or critical parts of oneself until some future date when scientists and doctors would have learned how to thaw you out and save you.

Some folks are still having themselves or their heads frozen to this day[iii] after they die. Cryogenics was most famously parodied in the very funny Woody Allen movie, *Sleeper*, in which Woody Allen's character is taken out of a frozen state in a dystopian future. The scene where he is unwrapped from aluminum foil like some kind of giant TV dinner is priceless.

It turns out that while many people still think cryogenics is largely a waste of time and money (not to mention being very weird), cryogenically preserving stem cells from your body is going more mainstream. Apparently it is starting to make sense to a growing number of people and governments to freeze stem cells. For others, it remains controversial. Whether one supports it or not at the present time, stem cell banking is a rapidly expanding, profitable business as well.

In stem cell banking you "deposit" (i.e. store) some of your stem cells in a high-tech super-freezer that keeps them ultra cold, most often via liquid nitrogen (Figure 6.3). In that state, the cells are kind of "frozen" in time. They are in "stasis", still alive but essentially in a state of suspended animation in which they do not age. In theory such cells can remain viable in that state for decades.

The most accepted form of stem cell bank stores umbilical cord blood, a practice that has been going on for more than a dozen years. California, for example, has set up a public umbilical cord blood bank program managed from here at UC Davis School of Medicine.[iv] I am not involved in that effort, but it sounds interesting to me. As discussed in Chapter 2, umbilical cord blood is rich in a unique type of stem cells that is thought to have great therapeutic potential.

[iii]http://www.nytimes.com/2002/12/21/sports/baseball-williams-children-agree-to-keep-their-father-frozen.html
[iv]http://www.ucdavisstemcell.org/cgi-bin/page.asp?sid=8&hid=19&id=

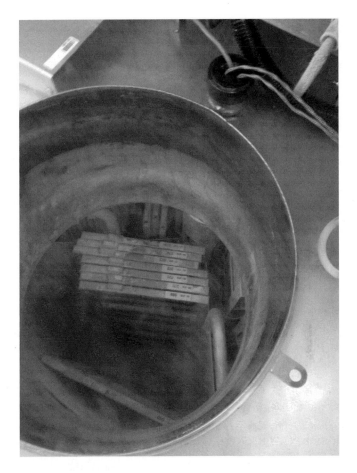

Figure 6.3. A human stem cell banking apparatus. The view is down into a liquid nitrogen tank. The wires near the top are from probes that monitor the temperatures at different levels in the tank. The inside of the tank is akin to a merry-ground as technicians can rotate it to retrieve a specific container of stem cells for a given patient. Racks of cassette boxes each containing 81 cryovials (up to 4.5ml of stem cells each) are visible.

What types of stem cells are banked?

Beyond cord blood, the most commonly banked stem cells are certain types of "adult" stem cells isolated from adipose tissue or bone marrow. Some folks have even advocated banking fibroblasts from skin, that general type of cell that can be made into iPS cells at some future point when clinically appropriate iPS cell production methods are perfected. Others have advocated banking the iPS cells themselves. There is considerable debate about whether it makes sense at this time to be banking one's stem cells.

The cases for and against stem cell banking

The case in favor of banking

Younger stem cells are better.

If you deposited cells in such a bank at age 30, over the next 3 decades you as a person would age to 60 years old and the endogenous stem cells in your body would be that "old". In contrast, your frozen stem cells would in theory not have aged and would remain with the qualities of your long gone 30-year old self if thawed and used to treat you. One can see how this might be medically useful either because of the youthfulness of the frozen stem cells or because later on in life you had some disease such as a blood cancer, which contaminated your endogenous hematopoietic stem cells in your bone marrow with tumor cells. The pure, relatively "young" frozen stem cells of yours could be thawed and used as the basis for a stem cell treatment for you later in life.

In addition to for-profit efforts, there continue to be academic programs to establish and maintain stem cell banks. In March of 2013, for example, CIRM issued more than $30 million for 9 grants related to banking of healthy and diseased stem cells including iPS cells.[v] The two largest grants went to the for-profit Cellular Dynamics International and the non-profit Coriell Institute for Medical Research ($16 million and nearly $10 million, respectively). The efforts for establishing as well as the potential pros and cons of iPS cell banks were also discussed in Chapter 2.

---

[v]http://www.cirm.ca.gov/about-cirm/newsroom/press-releases/03192013/stem-cell-agency-banks-32-million-new-approach-advance

The potential case against banking

One of the main arguments against banking can predominantly be summed up by an open question: how well do frozen stem cells really hold up over time periods that might span decades?

We do not know for sure how specific stem cells will hold up over decades in liquid nitrogen at commercial facilities. There are many variables including the relative health of the cells to start with, how they were frozen, and the temperature at which they are stored.

As a cell biologist I would predict that the stem cells cryopreserved that way for 20 or 30 years would not be quite as robust as they were when fresh. However, there is evidence the cells do well enough to be very clinically useful after such prolonged cryopreservation. For example hematopoietic stem cells and other progenitors cryopreserved for close to or even more than 20 years remain viable and functional [11, 12]. Human blastocysts cryopreserved for eighteen years were still able to produce pluripotent embryonic stem cell lines [13].

Over time with increased banking we will learn more about how the cells hold up and how to improve that efficiency. Opponents of stem cell banking argue that until we learn more, it would be premature to bank one's stem cells at this time.

It is also not entirely clear how the aged human body, say after twenty years, would react to an infusion of its own *Rip Van Winkle* stem cells, but there is no direct evidence that cryogenically preserved cells would illicit an immune reaction, for example any more than fresh ones as long as they were preserved prior to freezing without addition of xenoproteins such as those present in FBS. The levels of the cryopreservative DMSO that are used should not be too high either. When it comes to DMSO, 5-10% is considered acceptable.

Another concern about stem cell banking is cost.

One of the biggest challenges of stem cell banking from a potential patient's perspective is financial. Cell banks charge an upfront fee of up to a couple thousand dollars at the beginning and a yearly fee of up to a few hundred dollars to maintain the storage. It can really add up over time. However, proponents argue that it is hard to put a price on something that could be a life-saving therapy later on, for oneself or one's child.

Each individual person will have to decide if banking makes sense for him or her as a potential medical reserve for the future relative to the cost. Based on current trends, it would seem that more and more people are deciding that stem cell banking makes sense.

At the same time, banking technology methods are likely to improve over time as well in the future including such steps as advancing cryopreservation technology. It is a Catch-22 situation of sorts. If you wait to bank your stem cells until some future date, the methods are likely to improve yielding healthier cells. However at the same time your endogenous stem cells are getting older and fewer in number inside of you as you age. Every day they are exposed to more environmental insults, yielding most likely inferior cells over time. There may also be tipping points past which you can no longer easily get very many healthy stem cells. In addition, should you become sick with certain types of metastatic cancer or autoimmune disease prior to banking your stem cells, it may be too late at that point.

Bottom line on banking

Cryogenically preserving your stem cells may be something that more and more people around the world decide makes sense for them. I still have not banked any stem cells myself, but I can understand why some people choose to do it and I see it as an industry with tremendous growth potential because there is an inherent logic to doing it if the price is not overwhelming to you.

Summary

While there are to my knowledge no real stem cell anti-aging therapies today, I do have hope that in the future the lessons that stem cells have to teach us may in turn lead to bona fide medicines to battle aging. If the stem cell theory of aging proposed in this chapter is correct, for example, then drug-based approaches to maintain populations of healthy stem cells might increase human lifespan. Whether stem cell banking proves to be another cost-effective way to live long, healthier lives remains unclear at this time, but at least in principle it seems to me to have promise if individuals and society can bear the associated costs. At the same time unhealthy aging itself costs all of us greatly of course in intangible ways as well as more concrete ways such as in trillions of dollars in health care costs. I am excited to see what the future brings for the impact of stem cells on aging.

References

1. Signer, RASJ Morrison (2013) Mechanisms that Regulate Stem Cell Aging and Life Span. *Cell Stem Cell*. **12**:2:152-65.
2. Morrison, SJ, et al. (1996) The aging of hematopoietic stem cells. *Nat Med*. **2**:9:1011-6.
3. Nishimura, EK, SR GranterDE Fisher (2005) Mechanisms of hair graying: incomplete melanocyte stem cell maintenance in the niche. *Science*. **307**:5710:720-4.
4. Conboy, IM, et al. (2005) Rejuvenation of aged progenitor cells by exposure to a young systemic environment. *Nature*. **433**:7027:760-4.
5. Kuhn, HG, H Dickinson-AnsonFH Gage (1996) Neurogenesis in the dentate gyrus of the adult rat: age-related decrease of neuronal progenitor proliferation. *The Journal of neuroscience: the official journal of the Society for Neuroscience*. **16**:6:2027-33.
6. Blackmore, DG, et al. (2009) Exercise increases neural stem cell number in a growth hormone-dependent manner, augmenting the regenerative response in aged mice. *Stem Cells*. **27**:8:2044-52.
7. Macaluso, FKH Myburgh (2012) Current evidence that exercise can increase the number of adult stem cells. *Journal of muscle research and cell motility*. **33**:3-4:187-98.
8. Blasco, MA (2005) Telomeres and human disease: ageing, cancer and beyond. *Nature reviews. Genetics*. **6**:8:611-22.
9. Cao, HRA Hegele (2003) LMNA is mutated in Hutchinson-Gilford progeria (MIM 176670) but not in Wiedemann-Rautenstrauch progeroid syndrome (MIM 264090). *Journal of human genetics*. **48**:5:271-4.
10. Pichierri, P, et al. (2001) Werner's syndrome protein is required for correct recovery after replication arrest and DNA damage induced in S-phase of cell cycle. *Molecular biology of the cell*. **12**:8:2412-21.
11. Veeraputhiran, M, et al. (2010) Viability and engraftment of hematopoietic progenitor cells after long-term cryopreservation: effect of diagnosis and percentage dimethyl sulfoxide concentration. *Cytotherapy*. **12**:6:764-6.

12. Broxmeyer, HE, et al. (2011) Hematopoietic stem/progenitor cells, generation of induced pluripotent stem cells, and isolation of endothelial progenitors from 21- to 23.5-year cryopreserved cord blood. *Blood.* **117**:18:4773-7.
13. Pruksananonda, K, et al. (2012) Eighteen-year cryopreservation does not negatively affect the pluripotency of human embryos: evidence from embryonic stem cell derivation. *BioResearch open access.* **1**:4:166-73.

Chapter 7

Law and Order Stem Cells

While stem cells have great promise for both medical applications and theoretically for future approaches such as slowing aging, relatively speaking we (meaning scientists, doctors, and society) are still somewhere in the beginning phase of the stem cell revolution. As with any revolution, sometimes in the heady, passionate early phase there can be not just practical, but also legal challenges that arise. Hype can prevail. People can get used or hurt. There is a certain danger.

On the other hand we do not want to suppress innovation, which can interfere with the revolution. It would seem that a balancing act is required for the stem cell revolution. In this chapter I address the current evolving status of US federal laws and regulations on stem cell procedures. I also discuss the dilemmas facing the stem cell field as it increasingly becomes commercialized.

US Laws and Regulations on Stem Cell Procedures

What is the current law in the US that applies to stem cell procedures?

There are two main laws in the US that are directly relevant: the *Federal Food, Drug, and Cosmetic (FDC) Act*[i] and the *Public Health Service (PHS) Act*. These are long, complex laws, but there are some key sections that have great significance for the stem cell field that I can boil down for you into regular English. Most significantly, these Acts give the FDA authority to regulate biological products of certain kinds

---

[i]http://epw.senate.gov/FDA_001.pdf

including human stem cells. Therefore, barring a federal court specifically overturning a particular FDA decision, FDA regulations are essentially law when it comes to stem cells in the US. The FDA is given certain authority over stem cell biological products and procedures more specifically under several regulations including "21 CFR Part 1271.10"[ii] and "21 CFR 1271.15".[iii]

Courts can challenge how the FDA interprets regulations or the regulations themselves. While courts give great deference to FDA rules, it is always possible that a particular FDA regulatory framework could exceed the FDA's statutory authority, as determined by the courts. The process whereby courts could change the FDA framework may be initiated when a corporation that disagrees with a specific FDA regulation files suit.

Are Stem Cells a Drug?

The answer to the question of whether stem cells given to patients as a transplant are a drug is more complicated than you might think. The answer in part depends on not only what the product is and how it is manipulated, but also on both how and when the physician uses it for a medical procedure. The answer can be, depending on circumstances, "yes", "no", or even "maybe."

Generally, however, if the cells are grown in a lab prior to the transplant, the FDA says, "yes, they are a drug", while some others including some physicians wanting to do such transplants and some of their patients more often want the answer to be, "no".

What exactly are the options for regulating such laboratory grown or even non-laboratory grown stem cells beyond the simple "yes" or "no" debate described above? Stem cell therapies can be defined as therapeutics in two main ways.

First, subject to less regulation, stem cell therapies can be defined as so-called human cell and tissue products (HCT/P) that are "minimally manipulated". In this case, the colloquial term used to define such a stem

---

[ii]http://www.accessdata.fda.gov/scripts/cdrh/cfdocs/cfcfr/CFRSearch.cfm?CFRPart=1271
[iii]http://www.accessdata.fda.gov/scripts/cdrh/cfdocs/cfcfr/CFRSearch.cfm?fr=1271.15

cell product would be to call it a "361". Stem cell clinics generally want their products to be defined as 361 because those are subject to far less regulatory oversight.

Second, a given stem cell therapy can be defined as a biological drug termed a "351" by the FDA. Some stem cell clinics try to avoid a 351 definition of their product by the FDA. They want to steer clear of the 351 definition because it requires them (appropriately in my opinion) to conduct clinical studies and go through much more thorough pre-marketing approval from the FDA. Interestingly, some patients oppose the 351 designation for propagated stem cell therapies too because they believe that it impedes their access to novel stem cell treatments.

A third definition of sorts would be to consider a stem cell procedure to be the "practice of medicine", a term referring to part of the care that a physician provides a patient that is almost entirely outside the regulatory domain of the FDA and is overseen by state medical boards.

Another key factor is whether the stem cell product is employed medically as "homologous use" (meaning used in an equivalent way to the functions that the cells performed endogenously in the body) or not. Non-homologous use is another way to trigger a higher degree of regulatory oversight via the 351 designation being applied. For example, fat stem cells being used to treat Multiple Sclerosis, a neurological disorder, would be non-homologous.

Adding another layer of complexity is *when* the product is used. A stem cell product that is transplanted within the context of the same surgical procedure during which it was isolated, under section (b) of the 21 CFR 1271.15 regulation (e.g. a surgeon isolates fat from a patient during surgery and after some minimal manipulation transplants it back to the same patient while they are still there) is subject to less regulatory oversight.

At the present time, the FDA regulates cell therapy products that are "more than minimally manipulated" as 351 drugs.[iv,v] While the definition

---

[iv] http://www.fda.gov/BiologicsBloodVaccines/GuidanceComplianceRegulatoryInformation/Guidances/Tissue/ucm073366.htm
[v] http://www.fda.gov/BiologicsBloodVaccines/GuidanceComplianceRegulatoryInformation/Guidances/Tissue/default.htm

of the term "more than minimally manipulated" is complex, one seemingly unambiguous way to trigger having the FDA define a stem cell product as a 351 is by growing the cells in the lab. Current FDA guidelines define lab-propagated stem cell products as drugs (underlined emphasis mine):[vi]

> FDA currently views, for the most part, that somatic cell therapy products include the cell therapies as explained in the Federal Register Notice (Vol. 58 No. 197, 10/14/1993, p53248), "Application of Current Statutory Authorities to Human Somatic Cell Therapy Products and Gene Therapy Products". These cell therapies do not fit the 21 CFR Part 1271.10 criteria for regulation solely under section 361 of the PHS Act and are regulated as biological products subject to pre-market review and licensure. Human somatic cell therapy products include autologous or allogeneic cells that have been propagated, expanded, pharmacologically treated, or otherwise altered in biological characteristics ex vivo to be administered to humans and applicable to the prevention, treatment, cure, diagnosis, or mitigation of disease or injuries.

While the language of this FDA regulation is admittedly hard to fathom on first read, what it is saying is that laboratory-grown stem cells are not 361s, but rather are drugs (351s).

What this means is that to be compliant, companies today intending to sell such laboratory-expanded stem cell products to patients with the intention of transplantation must first go through much the same process as any company intending to develop and sell a chemical drug.

This FDA regulation is being challenged both in court and by the way some stem cell clinics are operating. As a result, the definition of a particular stem cell product or procedure as a 351 versus 361 could change in the future. Unlike individual laws, specific regulations can and

---

[vi]http://www.fda.gov/BiologicsBloodVaccines/GuidanceComplianceRegulatoryInformation/EstablishmentRegistration/TissueEstablishmentRegistration/ucm146772.htm

do evolve without necessarily being overturned and replaced by a new regulation, sometimes changing in significant ways over time. Two cases here in the US are particularly instructive in this regard and provide important background.

First, a company called Regenerative Sciences, Inc. (RSI) reportedly began offering a laboratory-propagated stem cell product to patients about five years ago [1]. The product was described as an autologous stem cell-based therapy that was expanded in a lab prior to transplant. The FDA defined the stem cell product as a drug, issued an injunction [1], and the parties ended up in court. Dr. Centeno of RSI described his perspective on the events that preceded the case ending up in court on my blog.[vii]

A major ruling was issued in the case in 2012 in which a US federal court ruled in favor of the FDA [2]. The ultimate fate of this litigation has not been decided as it is being appealed by RSI, but as of today in 2013 propagated stem cell products intended for transplant are drugs.

The second case, involving a Texas-based stem cell company called Celltex, is also still evolving. Starting operations in 2011, Celltex is a relatively newcomer to the stem cell world compared to RSI. It is perhaps most famous for being involved in the stem cell procedure done on Rick Perry. The Texas Governor received an autologous in vitro expanded stem cell transplant in 2011 during the Republican Presidential Primary Race in which he was a candidate. I met in person with Governor Perry in 2012 to discuss stem cell policy and he mentioned his stem cell procedure, which involved transplants of billions of autologous stem cell cells, in very glowing terms.[viii]

Arguably more significant in my opinion than Perry's experimental procedure is the fact that Celltex has in its relatively short existence developed laboratory amplified stem cell products, according to its own press releases, from approximately 230 patients.[ix] A significant number of these patients, perhaps nearly 100, have received actual transplants.

[vii]http://www.ipscell.com/2012/05/interviews-with-centeno-and-sipp-on-key-case-on-fda-authority-over-stem-cells/ includes the following excerpt:

[viii]http://www.ipscell.com/2012/06/meeting-with-texas-governor-perry-building-stem-cell-bridges/

[ix]http://www.bizjournals.com/houston/news/2012/12/19/celltex-files-restraining-order.html

In the original business model (for now at least no longer operative after an FDA warning letter to the company[x]), Celltex itself did not directly conduct stem cell transplants, but instead worked with separate entities here in the US. Independent clinics and doctors performed the actual transplants into the customers. While Celltex manufactured its stem cell-based product (via its past partner RNL Bio/Human Biostar Inc) and doctors continued to transplant the product into patients on a for-profit basis, the company apparently had not previously gone through the standard FDA drug approval process in advance. Celltex argued that it was not necessary since they believed that their stem cell product was not a drug. The FDA ultimately disagreed.

Perhaps drawing the FDA's attention to Celltex was a letter of concern about Celltex courageously sent to the FDA and made public by University of Minnesota Professor Leigh Turner. Shortly after that letter, in April 2012 the FDA audited Celltex and during that two-week visit the inspectors found quite a number of issues of concern. These FDA "observations" as the agency calls them (along with many subsections of more specific issues listed under the observations) were outlined in an inspection report called a "483" that has since come into the public domain.[xi] While the report outlined many concerns, perhaps most striking was that the FDA defined Celltex in the 483 as a "Drug Manufacturer" (Figure 7.1). This indicates that the FDA had determined that the Celltex stem cell product grown in culture was indeed a drug.

As mentioned above, later that year, the FDA warning letter led to a halt in Celltex-related patient transplants. While Celltex ran into federal issues with the FDA, it was not violating Texas state law at the time because to my knowledge there was no law directly pertaining to this area. It was only later that the Texas State Medical Board adopted regulations potentially allowing for such stem cell procedures [3, 4].

The Texas State Medical Board is one of the only medical boards in the nation to have any policy at all on stem cells for which it is to be commended, even if I disagree with that policy.

---

[x]http://www.fda.gov/ICECI/EnforcementActions/WarningLetters/2012/ucm323853.htm
[xi]http://www.ipscell.com/wp-content/uploads/2012/06/Celltex483.pdf

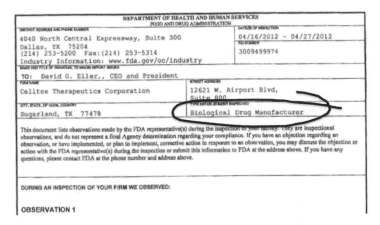

Figure 7.1. Top of the 2012 FDA 483 inspection report of Celltex indicating that in the FDA's view the company is a drug manufacturer, a definition that Celltex contested.

Surprisingly, more broadly it turns out that by federal law the FDA does not actually directly regulate physician conduct, but only drugs and medical devices. It is the job of state medical boards to oversee physician conduct. On first glance it may seem puzzling that most state medical boards lack policies on stem cell transplants, but one explanation is that a majority of states respect the federal jurisdiction in this area and the FDA guidelines. However, I would like to see state medical boards adopt rules that hold physicians accountable for their actions related to stem cell procedures.

What are the arguments against regulating propagated stem cells as drugs?

Some stem cell companies make the case that laboratory-expanded stem cell products should not be defined as drugs based on several arguments.

First, they assert that the amplification of adult stem cells in culture (prior to transplantation into patients) over a period of several weeks does not fundamentally change the nature of the cells. The claim that growth of stem cells in the laboratory does not substantially change the cells relative to the state of endogenous stem cells that are the starting material is flawed from my view (e.g. see "what can go wrong in the lab" in Chapter 5). Others clearly disagree and believe that allowing physicians to more readily transplant propagated stem cell products would help patients by making experimental treatments more readily available.

Second, ironically, some clinics claim that adult stem cell products meant for use in an autologous fashion "belong to the patient" and hence should not be subject to FDA regulation. This notion of patient ownership of their own cells, even if amplified into a stem cell product, is strongly promoted by some patient advocates for clinics too. I find this ironic because (as discussed in Chapter 9) in some cases it seems likely that patients give up their right to own their propagated stem cells, which are more likely to be owned by the clinics.

Finally, some clinics and their patient boosters argue more philosophically that regulating expanded stem cell products as drugs hinders innovation and slows the translation of stem cell therapies from the laboratory to the clinic. They assert that this regulation-related delay is harmful to patients. I am a strong believer in innovation, but my take is that rushing unproven stem cell procedures to patients may be more harmful to the patients than regulatory delays.

Balancing Innovation with Safety

Based on what we know today, laboratory-grown stem cells are different than endogenous stem cells in significant ways. In addition, their safety is not clearly established. Further, every lab that propagates stem cells for transplantation does it differently (sometimes varying in dramatic ways), making the risks of using the cells in patients in any one given clinical setting unclear.

A key larger question at the heart of this particular debate is how to best balance the objectives of promoting biomedical innovation and speeding new stem cell-based interventions to patients in need with the second goal of protecting those same patients from expensive, potentially unsafe, and ineffective stem cell-based interventions. I will discuss this question throughout the rest of this chapter as well as the ethical implications that arise.

While I favor regulation of lab-propagated stem cell products as biological "drugs" by the FDA at this time, you should be aware that stem cells are no ordinary drugs like pills. For example, if a patient takes a blood pressure medication and has a bad side effect, the patient can just stop taking the pills and within days the chemical ingredient in the medicine will disappear from the body naturally. However, in contrast, a stem cell drug (say consisting of a billion cells) is alive. Once injected, those cells move around the body and behave autonomously, particularly if transplanted IV.

What this means is that if patients have side effects after receiving stem cells, there is no way to remove the cells. In fact, while most transplanted stem cells die quickly, some of the stem cells may live and even grow inside the body, potentially for the lifetime of that patient. These attributes make stem cells very different from traditional chemical drugs, more unpredictable, and potentially far more dangerous. Given the capability of stem cells to cause unwanted tissue growth and because of their nature as living drugs, they pose unique and not entirely understood risks to patients.

Some patients facing devastating diseases for which today's medicine has no remedy understandably feel that the risk of trying an unproven stem cell intervention is at least worth considering. We cannot ignore their situation and I respect them, but at the same time the stem cell field should work toward more transparency by clinics and maintain our standards of expecting proven safety and efficacy for stem cell procedures. A rational, respectful debate over just how much regulation is ideal for both protecting patients and spurring stem cell-based innovation in medicine is healthy, but the debate over regulation of stem cell procedures often becomes heated and confused over such fundamental questions as:

How much regulatory oversight is appropriate versus too much?

What is the role of patients in deciding how much risk is acceptable?

What is the proper role of stem cell scientists, who generally avoid dealing with patients and for-profit operations?

How do we define a "legal" or "illegal" stem cell treatment?

I hope to convince you that an appropriate level of regulatory oversight of stem cell procedures is absolutely essential to protect patients and is compatible with innovation in medicine. A "Wild West", deregulated approach to stem cell procedures is a recipe for disaster. At the same time, I firmly believe that commercialization of stem cell products and procedures is necessary to move these therapies from the research lab to the clinic.

Compliant, but Scientifically and Medically Questionable Use of 361 Stem Cell Therapies

I also want to point out that laboratory propagation is not always an issue. Quite a number of companies offer stem cell procedures using cells that have not been more than minimally manipulated and are not grown in a lab prior to use. As described above, such stem cell products are called 361s (or may even qualify as "the practice of medicine", at least according to some physicians) and do not require quite the same intensive oversight by the FDA as do 351 stem cell drug products.

Companies in this category typically offer autologous, same day transplants of stem cells isolated from tissues such as adipose. Such stem cells can be rapidly prepared following liposuction or bone marrow isolation and re-injected into the same patient, who waits during that preparation. No growth of the stem cells in a lab is done and the adipose (or other) tissue cannot be treated with enzymes such as collagenase or mixed with exogenous growth factors.

While transplants of this kind are generally compliant with FDA regulations and most often pose a relatively low risk to patient, as a stem cell scientist I am highly skeptical that they actually help patients. The number of stem cells administered to patients is so low (typically in the low millions or less) that there is little chance of efficacy. In addition, if given IV, the body removes the cells so rapidly from the blood that there is minimal opportunity for the cells to do anything positive.

Even though the risk from such procedures is relatively low (but not absent), the likelihood of benefit is even lower. It is possible that future data will prove me wrong, but today, generally, I would say that such procedures are a waste of your money and not worth the risks (e.g. infection, unexpected immune response, etc) they do pose.

FDA Regulation of Stem Cell Claims

The FDA also is authorized by law to regulate product claims of medical businesses including those in the stem cell field. One of the most concerning aspects of the non-compliant stem cell field is that they make unsubstantiated claims about stem cell procedures, such as that they are risk-free and a panacea.

It is not uncommon to see a stem cell clinic website that lists almost every major disease known to humanity as treatable by them with stem cells. They falsely raise patient hopes with such bogus claims. Another claim made by stem cell clinics is that they will not just treat many diseases, but *cure* them using stem cells. I believe that in the future there will be specific diseases such as blindness that can be treated or even cured by stem cells, but we are not too close to that point today. The only stem cell cures out there are for blood disorders such as leukemias and immune system disorders.

The dubious stem cell clinics then have the gall to make the claim that they make no claims. It seems like something nonsensical out of *Alice in Wonderland*. In Figure 7.2 I depict the non-compliant stem cell snake oil salesman as a driver on a ramshackle advertisement-laden bus, making "no claims".

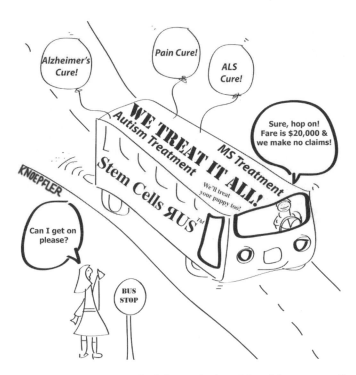

Figure 7.2. A depiction of a stem cell clinic on wheels making claims supposedly without making claims and a patient showing interest in getting help from them.

Human Subjects Research and IRBs

When patients are the subjects of research, they are called "human subjects". By law, the conduct of researchers who are doing studies involving human subjects must be overseen by a specific committee called an Institutional Review Board (IRB). The number one goal of IRBs is to protect patients, but from a dubious stem cell clinic perspective the number one goal of an IRB should be to approve their for-profit procedures and not impede them. One can see there is a clear conflict of motivations between some providers and IRBs.

In the US, IRBs are authorized at a federal level by the FDA, other governmental agencies, and federal regulations derived from the *National Research Act of 1974* to oversee research involving human subjects. As a result, IRBs have the power to approve or disapprove of research, or to require (for example, in the case of stem cell procedures) that a clinic or provider change their procedures in specific ways. IRBs also oversee human subjects research at universities as well.

Typically research institutions such as universities have their own internal IRBs, but a growing trend is the for-profit commercialization of IRBs. Commercial IRBs are generally faster than traditional institutional IRBs, which is a positive feature from the perspective of biomedical researchers and patients assuming strict standards are adhered to during review. However, others have raised concerns that some commercial IRBs may not be as exacting as institutional IRBs.

An FDA warning letter to the commercial provider of the Celltex IRB, Texas Applied Biomedical Services,[xii] raised concerns in the stem cell field. The FDA warning letter to this IRB provider (note it remains unknown if the concerns about the IRB provider had anything to do with its service to Celltex specifically) included concerns over failure to ensure members were free from conflicts of interest and the fact that the IRB apparently had no physician as a member.

The bottom line on IRBs is that they provide a key service to protect patients and stem cell procedure oversight by IRBs is generally a positive

---

[xii]http://www.fda.gov/ICECI/EnforcementActions/WarningLetters/2012/ucm323868.htm

thing, but not all IRBs are created equal and IRB-approval does not necessarily mean that a procedure is safe or effective.

Stem Cell Clinical Trials Process

The cornerstone of clinical research including that involving stem cell procedures is the clinical trials process. When a physician, a scientist or their organization wants to get FDA approval to test an innovative, laboratory propagated stem cell procedure in patients, they legally must go through the clinical trials process to determine, among other things, that the product is safe and effective.

How does this process work?

A preliminary consideration is determining whether what one is planning to do necessitates a clinical trial.

Today many doctors and clinics selling stem cell procedures argue that their procedures and the stem cells involved are exempt from the clinical trials process because the stem cells being used are not drugs. However, as discussed earlier the FDA views many kinds of stem cells (e.g. laboratory grown stem cells) used for procedures on patients as drugs that do require the clinical trials process.

A key foundation for stem cell clinical trials is a rigorous pre-clinical study of the stem cell procedure and the product involved. When administered in the same manner in which it would be given to human patients, does the stem cell drug show evidence of safety or efficacy in animal models such as rodents, dogs, or primates? What are its pharmacokinetics, meaning how does it behave in the bloodstream of animals? Is it toxic?

In the US, data answering such questions may be part of an Investigational New Drug (IND) application submitted to the FDA. If approved by the FDA, the company can proceed to start a Phase 0 or 1 clinical trial (Figure 7.3). The stem cell drug can also at that point be legally shipped across state lines. The IND application allows the FDA to evaluate preliminary pre-clinical data on the safety and efficacy of the new stem cell drug. The FDA specifies that the application "must contain information in three broad areas: Animal Pharmacology and Toxicology Studies, Manufacturing Information, and Clinical Protocols and Investigator Information."

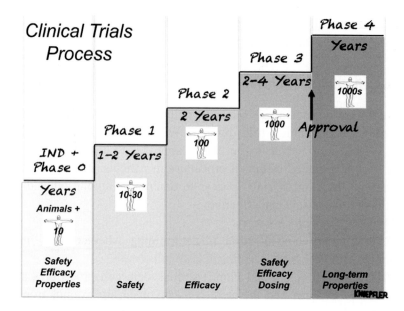

Figure 7.3. US Clinical Trials Process. Estimated time-line per phase is under the staircase, the number overlaid on the person symbol is the estimated range of the number of participants. At the bottom is the phase goal.

These requirements mean the IND application should (1) convince the FDA that there is a reasonable understanding of how the drug (in this case the biological drug in the form of stem cells) behaves in animals such as rodents or large animal models like pigs, dogs, or primates, (2) describe in detail for the FDA how the stem cell drug is made in terms of consistency, Good Manufacturing Practices (GMP), etc., and (3) explain how the company plans to study the drug in clinical trials.

In addition, because stem cells are no ordinary drugs, but are biological drugs, the company often needs to hold a specific license for that biological product before it proceeds, particularly if the stem cell product will cross state lines. In that case, a stem cell company must file a Biologics License Application (BLA) before touching a single patient. The BLA describes how the stem cell product is made and how it behaves in animals. Surprisingly, some clinics selling stem cell drugs to patients including patients from other states have entirely skipped the

IND and BLA processes.[xiii] However, I would stress that many stem cell for-profit companies are fully compliant.

Companies must present all this pre-clinical data to the FDA on safety and efficacy before doing anything with human patients. Then, with FDA approval, the team can start a Phase 0 clinical trial to study how the stem cell drug behaves in human patients. In a Phase 0 trial (that might have only 10 patients) as well as a Phase 1 trial (similar or slightly larger size), the main objectives are not to determine efficacy, but rather to understand how the stem cells behave and whether they are safe. For that reason, stem cells (as with any drug at this phase) are given at subtherapeutic doses, which lowers risks to patients as does keeping the number of patients enrolled rather minimal. The main distinguishing features of a Phase 0 trial from the Phase 1-3 trials is the minimal dose, the very low number of patients, and the goal of determining whether the drug behaves as expected. Note that Phase 0 trials are not always used.

If the results of the Phase 1 trial are encouraging, research can proceed to a Phase 2 trial (sometimes Phase 1 and Phase 2 are combined) involving more patients, which gives more robust data. Phase 3 trials typically involve hundreds to thousands of patients, which can lead to drug approval or rejection. It is worth noting that there are federal regulations intended to protect patients that specify whether and how companies can charge patients during clinical trials.

Ultimately, with evidence of safety and efficacy as well as a thorough understanding of how the drug behaves in vivo, the company may be permitted to sell the stem cell product after the trials. Phase 4 trials obtain data to optimize the use of the drug. Sometimes despite the rigorous evaluation of drugs prior to companies being permitted to sell them, certain significant side effects only become evident once the drug is used on many thousands of patients. What this means for stem cell procedures that are given to patients without any clinical trials or INDs at all is that their safety and efficacy are essentially a mystery.

[xiii]http://www.fda.gov/drugs/developmentapprovalprocess/howdrugsaredevelopedandappr oved/approvalapplications/investigationalnewdrugindapplication/default.htm

Suggestions for an Improved FDA of the Future

As much as I support the FDA's efforts to protect patients via employing regulatory mechanisms to promote safe and effective stem cell treatments (e.g. via the clinical trials process described above), it is not a perfect agency. In fact, certain aspects of the FDA actually are problematic for the field. To address these areas, I respectfully suggest (against the counsel of some colleagues who thought it too risky) five possible changes for the FDA moving forward (Figure 7.4).

(1) The FDA should work to partner with and guide those in the stem cell field who are pursuing innovation with good intentions. The FDA has a challenging relationship with many stem cell clinical researchers and physicians. One could reasonably say that in a number of cases that that is the fault of arrogant or simply clueless people who enter the clinical arena of stem cell-based medicine seeking to make money. I think that is true in many cases. However, in other cases there are people with good intentions who seek to commercialize stem cells and yet cannot seem to find a way to a healthy, productive working relationship with the FDA.

What is a potential solution here?

I believe the FDA needs to have a change in mindset. They need to find a more effective way to not just tolerate, but also actively promote innovation while protecting the safety of patients.

Proposed Changes to the FDA in the Stem Cell Arena

1. Promote innovation & a cooperative rather than antagonistic relationship with innovators
2. Accelerate and simplify decisions & regulations
3. Adopt a culture of greater openness
4. Take on a proactive approach
5. Facilitate patient access to trials and expand compassionate use of stem cells

---

Figure 7.4. Proposed changes to the FDA in the stem cell clinical field.

(2) The FDA needs to speed up and simplify. The FDA is too slow and complicated, problems it should remedy. The FDA has a very challenging mission that goes well beyond stem cells or other biological therapies so I think we need to understand that what they accomplish is remarkable. On the other hand, the FDA could be far faster and it could greatly streamline its approach to overseeing the development of stem cell therapies. I agree with the journal *Nature*, which said in a 2013 editorial that stem cell therapies need to be made easier [5]. Interestingly, the *Nature* editorial suggested that the delays at the FDA were linked to problems in the stem cell field such as stem cell tourism:

> "The longer it takes to develop a workable and affordable system in nations such as the United States, the more patients will travel for treatment to countries where there are even more unknowns."

I have spent considerable time reading FDA guidelines on their website. While I have learned a great deal through these efforts, I can tell you that it is a daunting challenge. The verbiage related to stem cell regulations is often dense, full of jargon, and generally difficult to understand even for a stem cell scientist. At times the language seems vague as well as leaving certain gray areas.

A first step to a solution for this issue is for the FDA to set goals for much faster turnaround times and accept that it needs to adopt a new communication style of clarity and simplicity. I can see no logical reason why FDA regulations have to be so difficult to understand. Policy documents should be written with an eye for clarity and ease of understanding.

(3) There is a compelling need for greater openness by the FDA with researchers, patients, study subjects, journalists, and concerned citizens. The FDA can be difficult to communicate with about stem cell issues. The FDA has a reputation for being somewhat inscrutable. People in the for-profit stem cell field tell me that they often find the FDA vague and unclear. Reporters who cover the stem cell field (incidentally reporters who cover science more generally are an increasingly endangered species) tell me that they frequently can get "nothing" out of the FDA. I myself have filed FOIA[xiv] requests with the FDA to try to get them to release documents faster. As it now stands it is not unusual for 6 months or more to pass after the FDA audits a stem cell clinic before that audit report is made public. That is far too long.

I have communicated with the FDA by phone and email several times. I found these interactions very helpful, but generally they will not go on the record about anything and have never explained to me why that is. I cannot quote them on my blog or in academic articles after such interactions. Patients tell me that they have trouble connecting with the FDA too.

I propose that the FDA work to have a higher degree of openness and accessibility. As much as it is understandable that the FDA needs to protect the intellectual property rights of companies and that it cannot discuss certain things (e.g. a clinic actively under investigation) necessitating some degree of privacy, I believe the FDA should revamp how it communicates to be more open and accessible.

(4) The FDA needs to be more proactive. The FDA is largely a reactive agency. It does not seem to stop problems very often before they escalate. Instead, too frequently, the FDA operates in a reactive mode. I call for a more proactive, anticipatory culture at the FDA. My sense is that the FDA largely waits for trouble in the stem cell field and then responds. I believe that they should take a more proactive approach instead. Part of their challenge is that they likely have limited resources and too few investigators. I have also recommended that the FDA needs more funding and staff to address these concerns.

It is relatively easy for my stem cell researcher colleagues and me to find non-compliant stem cell companies on the Internet. However, with few exceptions, the FDA takes no action against them unless they (1) get direct complaints from concerned citizens, (2) are contacted by concerned medical boards, or (3) if patients are harmed or killed and that knowledge enters the public domain. That must change.

[xiv] http://www.foia.gov/

It may be difficult for the FDA to monitor the world of dubious for-profit stem cell clinics in the US, but I understand from confidential sources that the FDA is aware of these clinics and that it does some level of screening for them. If in fact this is accurate, then I ask the following question: why is it that the FDA does not take a proactive approach with such non-compliant clinics and send investigators to inspect these facilities before patients are harmed?

The FDA needs to triage its actions when it comes to specific players in the stem cell for-profit field. Non-compliant companies that are putting patients at the highest risks by transplanting unlicensed laboratory grown stem cells (i.e. drugs) into patients should be subject to rapid action (as in months not years). Other clinics that are perhaps still bending if not breaking the rules should also be addressed, but perhaps with a lower priority. The current reality is that dangerous clinics may operate for years without any FDA action being taken to address the situation.

Being proactive may also mean auditing and contacting a putative non-compliant clinic to foster education and if possible a return to compliance.

(5) The FDA should make access to stem cell clinical trials easier for patients. One possible component of increased access would be expanding compassionate use to explicitly include very specific stem cell-based therapies. The *Nature* editorial mentioned earlier suggests this change as well and raises a few additional relevant points:

> "Certainly, there is room for the FDA to improve the regulation of stem cells. The large clinical trials that the rules currently demand are so expensive that many researchers and biotechnology companies cannot afford to conduct them. To ease that problem, the agency could explore expanding its 'compassionate use' clause, which allows individual patients to pay for drugs that are being used in FDA-approved trials. Alternative funding mechanisms, perhaps involving national insurance programmes, could be used to help offset the costs to patients and to those who perform the trials."

The FDA should make it easier for researchers trying to be compliant to get stem cell therapies that have some evidence of safety and efficacy to clinical trials for patients in need. Faster review would go a long way to improving the efficiency of the stem cell therapeutic pipeline. I have concerns about patients paying for compassionate use therapies though.

As a possible hint of change to come at the FDA in the arena of accelerating stem cell cures, the FDA held the first ever meeting on amyotrophic lateral sclerosis (ALS) in 2013, at which the wonderful stem cell advocate Ted Harada spoke.[xv] I hope that this meeting catalyzes real change, but I am not naïve enough to think that change will come easily to the FDA. In the past, the FDA has made statements indicating its intention to speed access to new therapies,[xvi,xvii] but so far patients tell me they have not seen much in the way of practical change in this regard.

Expanding Stem Cell Compassionate Use: Proceed, but with Caution

While I see the FDA as having a crucial role in the realization of the potential of future stem cell therapies, it is valuable here to discuss the issue of whether society has an ethical duty to allow terminally ill patients to choose to receive experimental stem cell procedures when all other options are exhausted through so-called "compassionate use".

Some of the patients who contact me have a disease or have a family member with a disease that has reached a point where they feel action is needed right away. I respect that and as a cancer patient myself I can understand that it is the patient who ultimately, with their physician, should make their own medical decisions.

[xv] http://www.alsa.org/news/archive/alsa-and-mda-urge-fda.html
[xvi] http://www.fda.gov/ForConsumers/ByAudience/ForPatientAdvocates/SpeedingAccesstoImportantNewTherapies/default.htm
[xvii] http://www.accessdata.fda.gov/scripts/cdrh/cfdocs/cfcfr/CFRSearch.cfm?CFRPart=314&showFR=1&subpartNode=21:5.0.1.1.4.8

It gets more complicated; however, when patients become interested in interventions (e.g. unlicensed stem cell procedures) that could do them great harm and negatively impact other patients as well as the whole stem cell field. Throw in the complexity of stem cell science and the disagreements even between physicians about certain issues, and it can be very difficult for patients to make informed decisions about the possible risks and benefits of such experiments procedures.

Some patients, especially those who advocate for specific for-profit, non-compliant stem cell clinics and doctors, often cite something called the Declaration of Helsinki[xviii] to argue for reduced regulation of stem cell procedures. The World Medical Association, an international medical body, has developed the Declaration to provide ethical guidelines for medical research on human subjects. It is notable that the American Medical Association has not wholly endorsed the Declaration and disagrees on certain issues.

Advocates of expanding the use of experimental stem cell interventions, especially for compassionate use, most often cite part 35 of the Declaration:

> "In the treatment of a patient, where proven interventions do not exist or have been ineffective, the physician, after seeking expert advice, with informed consent from the patient or a legally authorized representative, may use an unproven intervention if in the physician's judgement it offers hope of saving life, re-establishing health or alleviating suffering. Where possible, this intervention should be made the object of research, designed to evaluate its safety and efficacy. In all cases, new information should be recorded and, where appropriate, made publicly available."

This portion of the Declaration does not in fact promote the sale of non-compliant stem cell therapies to patients. Clinics selling such experimental procedures to patients also most often do not conduct or

---

[xviii]http://www.wma.net/en/30publications/10policies/b3/index.html

publish research. I would also argue that it is impossible for physicians charging patients for such procedures to avoid conflicts of interest and maintain a culture of putting the protection of patient rights first.

Compassionate use of stem cell interventions seems appropriate to me only in very specific cases where there is a medically demonstrable lack of other options for patients with terminal medical conditions. Under these conditions, I support it and believe the FDA should more explicitly define and allow for this to be more often employed in the US.

Why am I not even more enthusiastically supporting expansive compassionate use of experimental stem cell procedures? The risks of compassionate use going out-of-control are significant. Such dangers are illustrated by a chaotic situation in Italy[xix] in 2013. Italy has a more permissive biomedical regulatory climate relative to the US and many other parts of Europe.

In a battle played out largely in the media rather than within groups of physicians and scientists, the debate in Italy has been whether seriously ill patients can receive experimental stem cell procedures. The mainstream Italian media as well as some prominent Italian celebrities have weighed in on the side of allowing compassionate use of unproven, potentially even dangerous stem cell procedures.

Remarkably, Renato Balduzzi, the Italian Health Minister, decreed in March of 2013 that the unproven stem cell therapies in question should proceed for 32 terminally ill patients who are mostly children. According to the *Nature* piece, hundreds of protestors marched in the streets in favor of allowing the experimental procedures by a company called Stamina Foundation:

> "The unexpected decision on 21 March has horrified scientists, who consider the treatment to be dangerous because it has never been rigorously tested. In the opinion of stem-cell researcher Elena Cattaneo of the University of Milan: "It is alchemy".

[xix]http://www.nature.com/news/stem-cell-ruling-riles-researchers-1.12678

> The decision followed weeks of media pressure to authorize compassionate use of the therapy, which was developed by the Brescia-based Stamina Foundation and has been repeatedly banned in the past six years. Now, patient groups are pushing for the treatment to be available to anyone with an incurable illness. Hundreds protested in Rome on 23 March, including a naked woman with pro-Stamina slogans painted on her skin."

While there could be some justification of certain stem cell treatments for terminally ill patients in principle, it is not at all clear in this Italy case whether it is appropriate. To my knowledge there is little if any evidence demonstrating the safety and efficacy of the procedures in question. I also wonder in this case how one defines an "incurable" illness as opposed to a "terminal" illness? A serious overriding concern is that the stem cell therapies might literally kill the patients or make them even sicker.

The information in the *Nature* piece also points to another risk with out of control compassionate use of stem cells. This kind of media frenzy to promote procedures that are not evidence-based will most probably expand the use of such potentially dangerous treatments well beyond the compassionate use domain. The article quotes the president of the company Stamina as saying the publicity surrounding this situation has "won him 9,000 new patients". Presumably thousands of people not qualifying for compassionate use will nonetheless be given the same dubious stem cell therapy that lacks evidence of efficacy or safety.

The FDA needs more funding

Unfortunately, while the FDA has massive and growing responsibilities, it must handle these with a largely static budget (Figure 7.5). How can the FDA keep pace in this situation? I have called for an increase in FDA funding,[xx] but realistically in the messy budget times in the US, a boosted or even steady state FDA budget is unlikely.

[xx]http://www.ipscell.com/2012/09/as-stem-cell-industry-explodes-can-a-static-fda-keep-up/

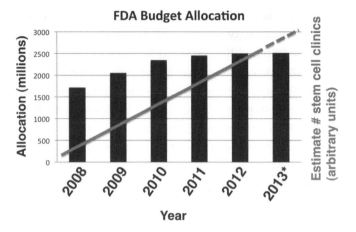

Figure 7.5. Estimated US FDA budget allocations by year sourced from FDA and Congressional budget documents (bars). The FDA budget is compared to my estimate of the relative number of stem cell clinics in the US (gray line, arbitrary units).

I believe the FDA should challenge itself to do more to address the five issues above with the resources that it already has. The changes suggested above could actually save the FDA money in the long run by reducing the need for punitive (and expensive) regulatory actions (and associated legal costs in some cases) in the stem cell field through greater openness and proactive solutions.

Summary

It will be fascinating to see how laws and regulations related to stem cell procedures continue to evolve over time both in the US and around the world. I do not expect the current (as of 2013) legal stem cell climate to remain unchanged in coming years. There could be significant loosening of the rules to, for example, allow for wider transplants of propagated stem cells or, alternatively, the FDA in the US could expand enforcement efforts and become more proactive in tackling the increasing number of noncompliant stem cell clinics. A change to allow more compassionate use in the US seems inevitable even if the timing of such a move is unpredictable.

The stem cell field must work to balance innovation and patient safety. Key factors to be aware of by all involved include the following: keep patient well-being at the forefront, be conscious of potential ethical pitfalls, maintain good-faith efforts to educate themselves and others, respect the law of the day even if one is working through legal means to challenge it, stay open to respectful dialogue with those with whom you disagree, and minimize secrecy on all sides.

Importantly, please note that medical decisions must be made with one's personal physician and no sections of this book are intended as medical advice.

References

1. Cyranoski, D (2010) FDA challenges stem-cell clinic. *Nature*. **466**:7309:909.
2. Cyranoski, D (2012) FDA's claims over stem cells upheld. *Nature*. **488**:7409:14.
3. DeFrancesco, L (2012) Texas legitimizes path around FDA oversight. *Nature biotechnology*. **30**:5:379.
4. Kaiser, J (2012) Stem cells. Texas Medical Board approves rules for controversial treatment. *Science*. **336**:6079:284.
5. (2013) Preventive therapy. *Nature*. **494**:7436:147-8.

Chapter 8

Stem Cells for Profit: An Ethical Spectrum

Stem cells saved a life.

Stem cells killed a baby.[i]

Both of the above statements are true, illustrating the power of stem cells equally to do good and harm.

In the case of the baby's death, it did not happen in some obscure, remote place in a ramshackle clinic, but astonishingly instead it happened at what was formerly[ii] the largest stem cell clinic in all of Europe called Xcell. The German Government has since closed Xcell down.[iii] In another case, a teenager died of a brain tumor caused by a stem cell procedure [1].

These tragic cases illustrate why stem cell procedures not only need to be effective, but also safe. In addition, they must be given to patients in an ethical manner by trained physicians.

What is an ethical stem cell treatment?

What are the key ethical dilemmas that arise during commercialization of stem cell interventions?

How can the stem cell field commercialize stem cell procedures without violating key ethical guidelines? I tackle these questions and challenging ethical issues in this chapter.

---

[i]http://www.telegraph.co.uk/news/worldnews/europe/germany/8082935/Baby-death-scandal-at-stem-cell-clinic-which-treats-hundreds-of-British-patients-a-year.html

[ii]http://www.telegraph.co.uk/news/worldnews/europe/germany/8500233/Europes-largest-stem-cell-clinic-shut-down-after-death-of-baby.html

[iii]http://blogs.nature.com/news/2011/05/notorious_stem_cell_therapy_ce_1.html

I do not want to give the impression that all stem cell companies are unethical rogues. On the contrary, some are doing great, innovative things in an ethical manner so below I start the chapter focusing on the positive of the good citizens of the field. Later I also explore the outright outrageous ethical breaches that some elements of the stem cell for-profit field are engaging in all too frequently.

Having Our Innovation and Ethics Too

In the stem cell field you can have it both ways. You can be ethical and help patients in an innovative manner. There are many examples of stem cell-related corporations doing "the right thing" when it comes to developing therapies based on growing stem cells in the lab. Below I discuss a few examples of these "good citizen" companies, although this list is of course not all inclusive.[iv]

Advanced Cell Technology

As one example, let me mention a company called "Advanced Cell Technology". ACT's most advanced product in the pipeline toward the clinic is an embryonic stem cell-based therapy for macular degeneration, the leading cause of blindness. ACT grows the embryonic stem cells in culture and differentiates them through a complex process into special cells called retinal pigmented epithelial cells (RPEs). Macular degeneration robs people of their sight because their endogenous RPEs die off. Therefore, the principle behind ACT's therapy is to replace the endogenous RPEs with exogenous ones, a cell therapy approach. So far, ACT has reported no major negative outcomes from its early trials of transplants of embryonic stem cell produced-RPEs. I discuss ACT here because it follows FDA rules and works in an ethical manner to protect patients. It publishes its data and engages patients.

[iv]Disclosure: I have no financial interests in these companies, which are listed in alphabetical order.

Athersys

Athersys is an adult stem cell company developing allogeneic products to treat a number of important human diseases. The company has five clinical trials listed in the government database.[v] The target medical conditions include stroke, heart attack, blood cancers, obesity, and ulcerative colitis. Their top-line product, MultiStem, is described by the company in one of their clinical trial write-ups as follows:

> "MultiStem(r) is a new biological product, manufactured from human stem cells obtained from adult bone marrow or other nonembryonic tissue sources. Factors expressed by MultiStem cells are believed to reduce inflammation and regulate immune system function, protect damaged or injured cells and tissue, promote formation of new blood vessels, and augment tissue repair and healing."

Athersys has a good reputation in the stem cell field for transparency including regularly publishing their data and following FDA regulations.

Mesoblast

Mesoblast is another good citizen in the stem cell field and has an unusually large number of stem cell products in the pipeline. Their work is based on a type of cell that they call the "Mesenchymal Progenitor Cell" or MPC. Interestingly, while typically progenitor cells have less potency than stem cells as we discussed earlier in this book, Mesoblast's MPCs are not your ordinary progenitor cells. I recently heard a talk by Dr. Paul Simmons of Mesoblast who reported that MPCs are in fact more potent than MSCs,[vi] which is an interesting paradox of nomenclature. Mesoblast is conducting FDA-approved clinical trials for a host of human diseases. I found nine clinical trials listed for Mesoblast including for conditions as variable as spinal disc injury and heart attacks.[vii]

---

[v]http://clinicaltrials.gov/ct2/results?term=athersys&Search=Search
[vi]http://www.ipscell.com/2013/03/viacyte-and-mesoblast-present-at-cirm-meeting/
[vii]http://clinicaltrials.gov/ct2/results?term=mesoblast&Search=Search

NeuralStem

NeuralStem is a fourth good citizen in the stem cell for-profit world. They are a model for the field when it comes to transparency,[viii] publishing data and even publicly releasing their patient consent form, a rarity in the biomedical for-profit world. NeuralStem currently has four clinical trials listed in the database: two on depression, one on spinal cord injury, and one on Amyotrophic Lateral Sclerosis (ALS; Lou Gehrig's Disease).[ix]

The key, positive roles of investors in good citizen companies

It is important to also highlight the crucial role of investors in making safe, effective, ethical, and compliant stem cell treatments a reality. For-profit stem cell companies including the good citizens of the corporate stem cell world need large amounts of cash to make stem cell-based medicine a reality.

The money comes from investors, who are hoping that some of the exciting stem cell biotech companies become profitable. I know from talking with many of the investors that they are choosing to invest in the stem cell companies not just because they believe that the companies will be profitable, but also because the stem cell products of those companies will potentially help people suffering from diseases and injuries. I believe that the investors in some publicly traded stem cell companies fulfill a key role in accelerating stem cell cures. The investors tend to be a highly educated, engaged group of people as evidenced by their posts on a website for stem cell investors[x] where I sometimes blog as well.

Investors in privately owned companies certainly can and do also have positive roles, but I am concerned that in that context the lack of transparency may predispose to a more complex, potentially ethically problematic influence in certain cases.

[viii]http://celltrials.info/2012/12/10/stem-cell-autopsy-neural-fetal-cell-persistence-als-trial/

[ix]http://clinicaltrials.gov/ct2/results?term=NeuralStem&Search=Search

[x]http://investorstemcell.com/

The main overall challenge in a for-profit setting is to create a business regulatory environment in the stem cell field that enables good actors to succeed.

Academic clinical researchers

There are also many academic centers working to produce safe and effective, ethical stem cell treatments. Generally they are highly compliant with FDA regulations in terms of production of stem cell therapies. Some of this inspiring, compliant research is going on right here at UC Davis School of Medicine in our Institute for Regenerative Cures,[xi] but there are dozens of other academic centers also doing great work without challenging the laws related to the clinical use of biological drugs or engaging in unethical conduct that endangers patients.

The Non-Compliant, For-Profit Stem Cell World

For some folks, the prospect of profiting from stem cell interventions lights up dollar signs in their eyes. Capitalizing on the excitement about stem cells, some entrepreneurs are already making big money offering stem cell procedures for diseases, injuries, and for aging itself. For the most part such stem cell procedures are not ready for prime time, yet these business people (who are often also physicians or working closely with physicians) are pushing the regulatory limit with the FDA and other regulatory agencies across the globe.

At the same time they challenge the FDA, some are likely fearful that they will get a knock on their door from the FBI because they know what they are doing is unethical, dangerous to patients and potentially illegal. What they may fear even more is a summons indicating that some of their patients are suing them for fraud or malpractice. I suspect other stem cell clinic operators and physicians are clueless. They do not even know enough about stem cells or applicable regulations to be fearful. A

[xi]http://www.ucdmc.ucdavis.edu/stemcellresearch/

common trend is for such non-compliant clinics to also engage in ethical abuses as well.

The patients who have chosen to go ahead and purchase stem cell transplants outside FDA-approved clinical trials are doing so even though the biomedical science has not proven them safe or effective. Some patients getting procedures at unlicensed clinics have admitted to me that they are knowingly very much human guinea pigs. They are paying for the privilege out of their own pockets to the tune of tens of thousands of dollars. Others incorrectly believe that the therapies are known to be safe and effective.

I wish the patients well, but I worry about the clinics taking advantage of the patients in their vulnerable state as well as taking money that patients and their family members cannot afford to lose. In many cases, the clinics providing the stem cell procedures aggressively market them to vulnerable patients and make false claims. These dubious stem cell clinics most often operate at the fringe, skirting regulation by the FDA and regulatory agencies in other countries. I will discuss the ethical problems of such clinics in the next sections. I have also included in the next chapter a practical guide for patients in evaluating possible stem cell procedures and a bill of rights for stem cell patients.

An Overview of Ethical Landmines in Stem Cell Commercialization

I recently gave a 2-hour presentation to trainees here at UC Davis School of Medicine who are involved in research and medicine in different capacities including physicians, graduate students, and medical students. We had a very interesting, dynamic discussion of the key issues involved in the ethical commercialization not only of stem cell therapies, but also innovative medical procedures and research overall. I took a picture of my white board after the talk because I thought it nicely captures the spectrum and complexity of issues involved (Figure 8.1). I will briefly go through the most compelling of these issues with you.

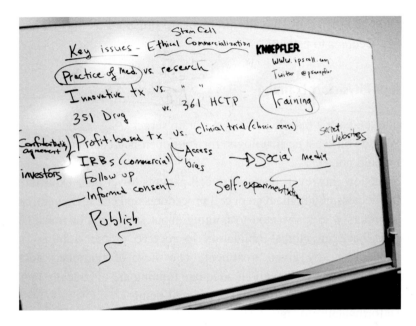

Figure 8.1. My white board after my lecture with trainees on ethical stem cell commercialization.

I started my lecture by arguing to the trainees the premise that commercialization of stem cell therapies, as with any innovative biomedical technology, is necessary.

The simple reason is money as mentioned earlier. Translating new medical technologies from the lab to the bedside where they can actually help patients requires typically at least tens of millions of dollars per new innovation if done in a compliant, ethical manner.

Non-profits acting alone most often are unable to translate technologies all the way through the entire clinic trials process to patients because they do not have that kind of cash, which instead comes from investors in privately held or publically traded for-profit companies with whom the non-profits form partnerships.

As much as commercialization is needed in the stem cell field, it raises certain ethical dilemmas and challenges that need careful consideration. A number of for-profit stem cell companies around the world have fallen into ethically problematic situations as they have sold their procedures to patients.

Lack of Physician Training

Would you have a radiologist do your brain surgery?

Would you see a dermatologist for your open-heart surgery?

I would not.

Somehow, however, many stem cell patients lower their expectations for the doctors giving them stem cell procedures and end up being treated by providers who know next to nothing about stem cells or transplants. Doctors have an ethical obligation to receive proper training prior to conducting any given treatment. The slew of untrained doctors transplanting stem cells without adequate training are unethically putting income as a higher priority than patient well-being.

Unfortunately to my knowledge there are no formal academic fellowship training programs for physicians in America to become specialists in stem cell-based cellular or regenerative medicine. Despite this training gap, individual physicians are still calling themselves "stem cell specialist", "regenerative medicine specialist" or "cellular medicine specialist". In essence they are using these pseudo-specialty claims to convince patients to come to their clinic without the specific, rigorous training needed to back it up.

I have proposed in a 2013 publication that medical schools and hospitals establish formal academic fellowship training programs in cellular and regenerative medicine [2]. In this way doctors could be properly trained (see components of my proposed curriculum in Figure 8.2) to conduct stem cell procedures. My hope is that patients would begin to expect the doctors at for-profit clinics to have real fellowship training in stem cells. Another objective is that the physician community would raise their expectations as well for stem cell training. Together these changes would lead to an overall substantial improvement in physician education and training in stem cells, lower patient risk, and improve compliance. In addition I hope that it would reduce regulatory actions by the FDA.

Proposed Stem Cell Fellowship Training for Doctors

1. Preclinical studies
2. GMP standards
3. MSC isolation and transplantation
4. Ethics
5. IRB issues
6. FDA regulations
7. Cell Biology
8. Patient rights
9. Emerging technologies

Figure 8.2. Proposed physician training program. Note that now physicians are not trained in any of these areas in medical school.

Interestingly, a cottage industry of supposed stem cell training for physicians has sprung up. After spending a weekend say golfing and attending a few hours of lectures, a doctor gets a fancy looking certificate to hang on their office wall that says they have been trained in stem cells. I am not sure what is worse about such "diplomas": their influence on patients or their impact on the doctor's own state of mind such that he or she actually believes that they are really qualified and properly trained to treat patients with stem cells. I have never myself been in a "stem cell doctor's" office, but both doctors and patients have told me about the pseudo-diplomas.

Another problem is the emergence of stem cell clinical preparation kits. One stem cell doctor in the business of doing transplants, complained to me about the problem of these stem cell purification kits because they enable essentially untrained doctors to get into the stem cell business and put patients at great risk. It is unclear how well the kits work and if their use would, from an FDA perspective, cross that significant line over to more than minimal manipulation to produce a stem cell drug. This would depend on the ingredients in the kits and how the kits are used. These troubling kits will be discussed further later in this chapter.

Stem Cell Tourism

Another major issue in the stem cell field raising critical ethical and safety issues is so-called "stem cell tourism", when patients travel from one state or country to others for stem cell procedures. Often this travel occurs because the stem cell clinic offering the procedure cannot legally conduct business in one country such as the US since the clinic is breaking the law or on the edge of doing so. As a result, the clinic sets up shop elsewhere. Some clinics sprout from day one outside the US and are owned by people in that country. Notably, in many other cases US citizens own stem cell clinics operated on foreign soil.

Stem cell tourism has been going on for at least ten years, but seems to have accelerated recently. Common destinations for American stem cell tourists include Mexico, Latin America, Germany and other European destinations, and Korea as well as other Asian countries. Stem cell tourism is also a common practice among people from countries other than the US. For example, many Europeans go to Asia for dubious stem cell treatments.

Stem cell tourism presents many potential problems and puts patients at greatly increased risk. Treating physicians almost uniformly are not giving stem cell tourist patients the proper follow-up needed at least in part because the patient and physician reside in different countries. Should anything go wrong with the procedure in a foreign country, the patient is at higher risk of additional, severe complications. It also is unclear whether stem cell tourists, should they have side effects or otherwise feel they were harmed by a physician in another country have any legal recourse. Other countries have very different, perhaps in some cases even dysfunctional legal systems compared to the US. There are also language issues and many countries surprisingly have no tradition of or laws regarding medical malpractice.

Dubious stem cell companies on the international market also have a way of disappearing or morphing over time into reborn companies with new names. Some of the proprietors also quite literally change their own personal names or go by aliases. Together these factors increase risk further for patients engaging in stem cell tourism.

The ISSCR has developed some questions that patients should ask regarding clinics in other countries [3]:[xii]

- Is the treatment routine for the patient's specific disease or condition?
- What are the possible benefits to be expected, how will they be measured, and how long will it take to see results?
- What is the scientific evidence that the treatment will work and where was it published?
- What are the risks of the procedure itself and possible adverse effects?
- Is there an independent body, such as an institutional review board, to oversee the treatment plan?
- Does a national or regional regulatory agency, such as the US Food and Drug Administration (FDA) or the European Medicines Agency, approve this treatment of this specific disease?

Stem cell tourism is a truly international concern and many articles have been written about it from the perspectives of numerous countries besides the US including Canada [4], India and Japan [5], and the UK [6].

The bottom line is that stem cell tourism greatly increases risks for patients. Some stem cell tourists have never returned home at all as they have died, while others have returned home and died there. A stem cell tourist cannot realistically expect to be treated in an ethical, safe manner.

Stem Cells Go Global

Another major, related issue in the stem cell field is that many firms increasingly are doing business in multiple countries. Some operate simultaneously in multiple countries. Others move from country to country, usually following a path of least resistance at the regulatory level. In the case of the former German stem cell company, Xcell, its

---

[xii]http://www.closerlookatstemcells.org/

leadership has now opened a new stem cell clinic in Lebanon since Xcell was shut down by the German government.[xiii]

Perhaps not surprisingly, the increasingly international nature of the stem cell industry (including legitimate and dubious players) has sparked emerging legal and ethical issues. In addition, the global nature of the stem cell for-profit world raises concerns related to the transport of stem cell-based biological drugs across international borders.

Think you can just FedEx human stem cells anywhere you want in the world? Think again. Transport of human stem cell materials across international borders is an exceedingly complex task if done lawfully and ethically.

Companies thinking of shipping their human biological drugs, such as stem cells, across international borders have a slew of governmental agencies that they must deal with in order for the export/import to be legal. In additions to Customs, in the US just two of the agencies are the FDA and CDC. It is not a simple matter, illustrated by the 61-page set of guidelines just from the FDA on export of biologics.[xiv] I am not an expert in this area, but a glance at this document suggests companies need FDA approval to export biologics/drug products.

The case of the Korean stem cell firm RNL Bio, which also does business in the US via subsidiary companies called Human Biostar and RNL Biostar, is notable. RNL is reportedly[xv] under investigation by the Korean government for alleged smuggling of stem cells from Korea across the border into Japan and/or China. A *Korea Times* piece mentioned a response by RNL to this allegation:

> "RNL Bio claimed the current law requiring researchers
> to receive certification for stem cell treatments after
> undergoing three rounds of clinical testing was a
> violation of the right to conduct research.

[xiii]http://www.telegraph.co.uk/health/healthnews/9192216/Stem-cell-doctor-forced-to-close-his-clinic-after-childs-death-is-back-in-business.html
[xiv]http://www.fda.gov/downloads/RegulatoryInformation/Guidances/ucm125898.pdf
[xv]http://www.koreatimes.co.kr/www/news/nation/2013/01/116_128264.html,
http://news.asiaone.com/News/Latest%2BNews/Health/Story/A1Story20121225-391519.html, and
http://english.chosun.com/site/data/html_dir/2012/12/24/2012122401244.html

The prosecution plans to restart its investigation dependent on the ruling from the Constitutional Court. The company did not give an immediate response to whether the allegations were true, but said it would release a public statement today".

I have checked and been unable to find a press release by RNL on this issue and I also tried to contact the company by email, but received no response. RNL is of course innocent of all charges until or unless proven otherwise, but the case highlights the possible legal complexities of moving stem cells across international borders.

Given that stem cell drug products can cost patients tens of thousands of dollars and hence have substantial commercial value, an additional issue is whether there would be major costs such as tariffs or taxes associated with transborder shipment of the items.

Patients packing stem cells?

There are unsubstantiated rumors more generally that some companies have already had their patients take stem cells across international borders on their bodies or in luggage without any government approval. If true, this kind of practice is clearly unethical on the part of the stem cell companies. It would seem to put patients at legal risk should this be discovered and shift the legal risk away from the companies and to the patients, raising serious ethical issues. Such stem cells also have a high possibility of being biologically compromised during this form of cross border transit putting patients at additional, in this case medical risk.

Of course it is also possible that companies may simply FedEx or otherwise overnight ship cells on liquid nitrogen or dry ice without any governmental approvals at all, but eventually they are likely to get caught. I think this practice also puts patients at risk as samples could again be compromised.

The issue of international transport of human stem cells is likely to come even more to the forefront this year and the near future as more and more companies seek to transport human stem cells across international borders. For example, Texas stem cell company Celltex has recently announced that it plans to try to set up procedures for its patients in Mexico, but all of their stem cell patient samples are stored in the US. Interestingly, most of the Celltex patient samples are apparently currently still in possession of Human Biostar, a Texas subsidiary of the Korean company RNL Bio mentioned earlier.

How would the Celltex samples get across the border into Mexico? Would the FDA or Customs or other agencies have to be involved and would they allow it? It is unclear whether anybody knows. I queried Celltex about the plan for Mexico-based procedures, but they had no comment prior to my press time for this book.

Call It Anything but Research: Avoiding Regulation

A fierce debate is taking place on the Internet and in the courts over how new stem cell therapies should be classified and named. It turns out that the way one defines and names an evolving medical therapy is not just a matter of semantics, but has major legal implications. Many for-profit stem cell clinics want their medical interventions to be called anything but "research" because that term invokes a higher level of regulatory oversight. That oversight is needed to protect patients, but it tends to reduce profits for the clinics.

It seems logical to me that experimental, new medical therapies that are part of clinical research should be defined as "research". However, the physicians and clinics that are today selling such experimental therapies to patients, often for twenty-to-thirty thousand dollars a treatment, do not like the word "research" to describe what they are doing. If their work is "research" then it is held to a different standard and can be regulated by the FDA in a different, more time-consuming and costly way (think 351 versus 361 versus "the practice of medicine"). For example, for stem cell procedures that are classified as research, clinics must conduct clinical trials and obtain pre-marketing approval from the FDA.

Instead, the sellers of experimental stem cell therapies (and indeed other medical procedures more broadly well beyond the stem cell arena) prefer to use two other terminologies: "the practice of medicine" and "innovative procedures".

If a physician transplanting stem cell into a patient is technically just doing "the practice of medicine", they can at least try to tell the FDA to mind its own business and leave them alone.

Another semantic and legal tactic is to call a new experimental therapy not "research", but rather an "innovative treatment". Again, this may sound like linguistic jujitsu, however it has important regulatory implications as technically physicians can perform innovative procedures without the same kind of regulatory scrutiny that is required for "research".

To my way of thinking, injecting patients with billions of stem cells that have not been proven to be safe or effective, and seeing what happens is logically research that requires oversight by the FDA. It is notable that it is not just small for-profit companies, but also large research institutions that sometimes seek to have their biomedical research classified not as research.

Potentially Divided Loyalties: Profits Versus Patients

Paying to be a human Guinea pig

Some clinics may try to avoid the clinical trial process (described in the previous chapter) entirely by making arguments that they are just practicing medicine as mentioned above, but in most cases in the end they must perform clinical trials.

Not all clinical trials are the same. Traditionally, patients go into clinical trials realizing that they are research subjects. I think these people are often heroes. They might hope to benefit from the new medical procedure or drug being tested in the trial, but also many of them desire to contribute to society and help future patients through their participation. Other than participating in the trial, traditionally patients are not expected to contribute in any other way to it. However, it is now common practice in the non-compliant stem cell for-profit field to charge patients to be part of clinical trials.

In my view, the practice of charging patients tens of thousands of dollars to be research subjects injected with unproven stem cell therapies is unethical. This is not only my view, but also federal regulations place significant constraints on when companies can charge research participants while operating under an IND (Investigational New Drug) application. In most circumstances companies cannot charge research participants — and if they do charge they must first have approval from the FDA. Perhaps to sidestep these rules, many companies simply break the regulations and do not get an IND.

Charging patients huge sums of money also raises potential bias in such studies because the only subjects who will be able to participate are those that have the money. A moral question of access also comes up again because inevitably in such circumstances people in lower socioeconomic groups will be excluded and not have the opportunity to participate. One might say perhaps these patients are lucky to avoid such dubious procedures, but access is an important issue.

Charging for clinical trials also raises conflicts of interest for the clinic and physicians involved as they have a vested interest in having patients participate and in positive outcomes.

Priorities: Big-money investors over patients?

Another potential complication at an ethical level is that for-profit stem cell companies inherently will have conflicts of interest between a duty to their patients and a sense of responsibility to generate monetary returns for investors. This kind of conflict of interest manifests whether the for-profit business is privately held or publicly traded. Investors want to see results in the form of profits, a priority that may not always be in line with what is in the best interests of patients and potential future patients.

In the case of a publicly traded company doing stem cell procedures, the Israeli business Pluristem has come under scrutiny for allegedly having a propensity to announce good news, for example proclaiming in a press release that they saved a pediatric patient's life, while supposedly not reporting bad news such as patient deaths.[xvi] Bloomberg reporter David Wainer, reporting on the story, is a harsh critic of the company:

> "The flurry of press releases and lack of follow-up shows the pressure early-stage drug companies are under to generate investor excitement. As with most biotechnology companies that have no drugs on the market, raising money through stock sales is Pluristem's main way of financing product development."

I have no specific, first hand knowledge of the Pluristem case or whether the concerns about their conduct are genuine, and the company may be innocent of these charges. I raise the case to point out in a more general sense that public announcements (or lack thereof) by stem cell companies that make claims of safety or efficacy have the potential for powerful and at least in theory sometimes harmful effects.

For privately held for-profit companies the influence of investor expectations on company practices involving patients is less obvious, but still of great concern.

Another related issue is lack of proper follow up of patients, a topic covered in more depth in Chapter 9. Some stem cell clinics do not conduct proper follow up monitoring of their patients, compromising safety and impeding the dissemination of knowledge, perhaps simply because they find it too expensive. To do such follow up of patients might make a business model less attractive to investors.

Lack of Proper Informed Consent

Any time a patient receives a medical treatment, the treating physician is supposed to first give the patient specific information (e.g. risks and benefits of the procedure, risks of not having the procedure, conflicts of interest on the part of the physician, and so forth). Based on this

---

[xvi]http://www.bloomberg.com/news/2012-11-07/girl-dies-as-pluristem-sells-on-gains-with-miracle-cells.html

information, the now informed patient can consent (or not) prior to the physician doing the procedure.

Informed consent by patients is particularly essential for those receiving innovative therapies/drugs as part of experimental research because these are inherently higher risk situations for patients. As a result, physicians obtaining informed consent from patients for innovative stem cell therapies should be telling the patients in an accurate way that there are likely to be unknown risks involved, that there are also known risks, and that there is no rigorous scientific data yet proving a reasonable likelihood of benefits. However, you can imagine that giving such information as part of the consent process would be likely to scare away many patients, reducing the company's profit.

Perhaps for this reason, anecdotal evidence suggests that many non-compliant stem cell for-profit companies do not ensure there is proper informed consent. Risks are minimized and potential benefits are exaggerated, giving patients a skewed perspective. This unethical lack of proper informed consent, even absent any other concerns, technically means that many stem cell therapies may be administered illegally.

Self-Experimentation

A concerning trend in the for-profit stem cell field, but one that does not get enough attention is self-experimentation.

While there is a history in science of self-experimentation, I believe that in the stem cell field it is fraught with danger both to the people involved and to others who might have altered perceptions about stem cell interventions as a result.

Scientists who are self-experimenters sometimes are dubbed as brave heroes of a sort. For example, Dr. Barry Marshall experimented on himself by infecting himself with the bacterium *Helicobater pylori* to test the hypothesis that it causes stomach ulcers. He became somewhat of a scientific folk hero and went on to win the Nobel Prize for his work along with Dr. J. Robin Warren in 2005.[xvii]

[xvii]http://www.nobelprize.org/nobel_prizes/medicine/laureates/2005/press.html

However, there have been many disasters related to self-experimentation. I suspect few of these end up in the public domain so what is known about negative consequences from self-experimentation is probably just the tip of the iceberg of what has actually happened. Two examples come to mind that ended badly.

Dr. William Stark self-experimented on the relation between diet and scurvy, and in so doing accidentally killed himself.[xviii]

Dr. Jesse William Lazear experimented on himself while studying yellow fever resulting in his own death.[xix]

So when it comes to stem cells, you might ask, "What's so bad about stem cell self-experimentation of this kind?"

Beyond the danger to the physicians themselves, a more serious problem in my opinion is that self-experimentation is used as a way to promote unlicensed stem cell procedures to patients. I have talked to patients who say that when a stem cell doctor says to them, "I get these procedures myself" it can be powerfully persuasive. As an analogy, imagine both you and your doctor have high blood pressure and as your doctor is recommending a specific drug for this condition to you, she says, "I take this medicine too." That is not self-experimentation because the drug has been FDA approved and its use is not experimental, but the point is that a personal testimonial from a doctor to a patient about their own experience with a specific drug or procedure is going to convince many if not most patients to try it. I would find that very compelling.

In the stem cell field, self-experimentation manifests when leaders of for-profit stem cell companies very often publicize that they themselves have received large numbers of procedures using their own company's stem cell products.

Stem cell self-experimentation may also change the thinking of corporate leadership such that they themselves become more viscerally passionate about the stem cell therapies in question to the point of losing their perspective and endangering patients. Some in effect may become addicted to stem cell procedures (Figure 8.3).

[xviii]http://en.wikipedia.org/wiki/William_Stark_(physician)
[xix]http://en.wikipedia.org/wiki/Jesse_William_Lazear

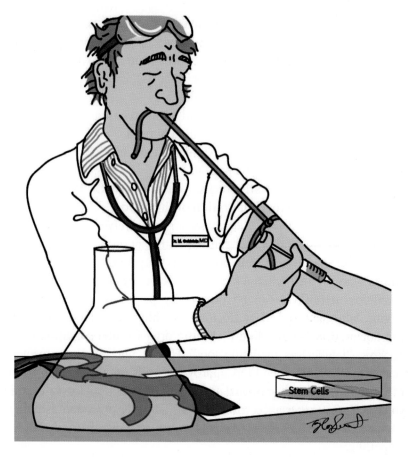

Figure 8.3. A hypothetical stem cell doctor self-experimenting. Illustration by Taylor Seamount.

Recruiter-Patients

Unfortunately, some patients get pulled into the world of dubious for-profit stem cell clinics and instead of advocating for other patients or for compliant research at good citizen companies, they advocate for for-profit, non-compliant clinics. Indeed, some patients who receive procedures from for-profit, dubious clinics become intensely aggressive advocates for those clinics. They encourage other patients to go to the same clinic. Through powerful video testimonials, blogs or other websites, these stem clinic patients often put in substantial effort to attract additional patients to the clinics. They become what are called "recruiter-patients", discussed in depth in an article about this common practice in India in the stem cell clinic world there [5].

I believe that in many cases these efforts by patients are genuinely motivated by their desire to help other patients because they believe (rightly or wrongly) that the clinic or doctor in question can provide helpful procedures to other patients suffering from the same disease. There is an understandable camaraderie between patients motivating such actions.

However, in other cases, it remains unclear whether some of the former patients are now secretly paid advocates for the clinics (e.g. perhaps getting discounts on future procedures or cash). As a result, it can be very difficult for patients considering whether or not to get a stem cell procedure for themselves or a loved one to know whom to trust and what is motivating people's advocacy of specific clinics.

My understanding is that there are patients who receive some kind of compensation for promoting clinics. In my opinion they are clearly betraying their fellow patients and potentially behaving in an unethical manner by not disclosing their compensation. It would seem like a form of fraud to me. The for-profit stem cell clinics are also betraying patients by using them as tools to increase profits.

Another Clinic Trick: Fake Patients as Recruiters

As discussed above, sometimes patients who have had experimental procedures done at dubious stem cell clinics become the biggest defenders of and advocates for those clinics. As I said, I believe that the vast majority of such clinic advocates are patients who simply believe strongly that the clinic helped them and want to convey that news to others. A minority may receive compensation from the stem cell clinic to make testimonials or to recommend the clinic to other patients on social media as discussed in the previous section.

Unfortunately, also in the mix are outright fake patients. They never received any procedures, but for a fee play the part of satisfied customers. In my mind these people and the clinics that pay them are exploiting the real patients as well as vulnerable potential future patients who are considering getting a stem cell treatment. Their actions may reasonably be called fraudulent. Confidential sources have informed me of fake patients, but to my knowledge there are no published academic or mainstream media articles on this potentially explosive topic.

Ethical Challenges in Stem Cell Social

In Chapter 1 I discussed some positive, helpful social media resources for readers to stay up to date on the stem cell field. However, there is another, darker side to stem cell social media. Many non-compliant stem cell businesses use social media to get new customers, often via ethically questionable practices, or to attack perceived critics.

While following the rapid increase in the number of dubious clinics over the years I have become familiar with their standard operating procedure (SOP) for marketing. Social media is a key element.

Stem cell facilitators endanger patients

The first step for unlicensed stem cell clinics is to stimulate cash flow. They need to find some way to attract clients so they try to generate some kind of publicity, but at the same time they face a paradox in that regard because too much publicity may attract unwanted FDA attention. Another paradox for dubious stem cell businesses is that the more patients they treat, which in theory is a good thing because it generates income, the more people there are who could sue them for stem cell fraud or malpractice.

Dubious clinics rely upon the strategy of funneling patients in their doors mostly via the Internet, sometimes via public websites and other times via secret websites (see Chapter 13). They use stem cell facilitators to help them drum up business.

What exactly is a stem cell facilitator? They are wolves in sheep's clothing. A typical stem cell facilitator might be a blogger or someone posing as a patient advocate. Via websites they hype stem cell procedures, particularly at certain clinics. They direct patients to such clinics and doctors, and in exchange the prevailing opinion is that they get a "finder's fee" for each patient. It is difficult to know much about them since they operate partially in the shadows.

Dubious clinics usually establish a website that promotes their clinic, often making unsupported claims of efficacy and safety. They pay the stem cell facilitators to "talk up" their clinic on blogs and on patient message boards. Pretty soon clients start coming in and cash starts to flow.

It remains unclear the degree to which the FDA has the manpower to monitor the Internet for the increasing number of websites of dubious stem cell clinics in the US making potentially unwarranted claims or selling unregulated stem cell procedures. Clinics generally are counting on the vastness of the Internet and the ever-growing universe of stem cell clinics to limit the likelihood that the FDA will investigate them specifically. It would seem to me that the FDA should view stem cell facilitators as putting patients at particularly high risk since the facilitators are causing relatively high numbers of patients to be put at risk, but would the FDA have jurisdiction to pull in the FBI to go after facilitators? It is not clear.

Recruitment of clients to other countries via social media and the internet

Another strategy of non-compliant stem cell clinics with possible regulatory issues is to attract clientele from the US, but to not actually operate a clinic in the US. Instead, they might have their clinic in Latin America or Asia. The Caribbean, Mexico, Panama, Thailand, the Philippines, and China are all particular popular locations for dubious stem cell clinics. Their thinking may be that by operating outside the US, they reduce their liability. However, recently a federal lawsuit for alleged fraud related to stem cell procedures was filed in California against the Seoul Korea-based company, RNL Bio, suggesting that litigation can easily cross international borders.[xx]

[xx]http://www.healthintheglobalvillage.com/2012/07/05/rnl-bio-jeong-chan-ra-human-biostar-inc-jin-han-hong-sued-for-fraud-in-stem-cell-lawsuit/

RNL Bio is innocent of any wrongdoing unless proven otherwise in court and it may well have done nothing wrong here (the case is still pending resolution). I mention the case only because it illustrates how patients can sue a company in US court related to stem cell procedures even if that company is headquartered outside the US and the procedure took place outside the US. If patient recruitment occurs in the US or if the patients are US residents (even if not citizens) in some cases it seems that a lawsuit can be filed against a non-American company.

Stem cell sockpuppets: Intimidation as a tactic to silence clinic critics

Proponents of for-profit adult stem cell procedures also often engage in a practice on the Internet called "sockpuppetry".[xxi] An Internet sock puppet is a person who assumes a false identity to sow confusion and launch anonymous attacks on others on the web. In the case of the stem cell world, proponents of adult stem cell therapies have launched regular sock puppet attacks on critics of unlicensed stem cell therapies. One of their favorite strategies is to adopt a fake Internet identity with a name similar to a critic's name to make inflammatory comments on stem cell-related news stories or use actual blogs to attack a particular critic.

The prototypic stem cell sock puppet's goal is to promote confusion and spread misinformation by pretending to be the real person in the stem cell field and making statements that are a jumble of inflammatory or even derogatory assertions. As a result stem cell scientists and patients as well as others in the field often get very confused. Sometimes patients are misled by the puppets to get angry with scientists.

Unfortunately I myself have developed several Internet sockpuppets who regularly attack me for being an advocate of regulatory oversight of stem cell experimental procedures and patient safety. It could be considered a compliment in a way if it means that they view me as influential enough to have to attempt to silence me. However, they have not and will not ever influence my actions and perspectives in the stem

---

[xxi]http://en.wikipedia.org/wiki/Sockpuppet_(Internet)

cell field. Their cowardly attacks only harden my resolve that patient safety and benefit should be the preeminent focuses in our field.

Strategic Lawsuits Against Public Participation (SLAPP)

Another tactic of intimidation against critics of the unlicensed, for-profit stem cell field is to threaten the advocates of regulatory oversight with lawsuits. Such lawsuits are termed strategic lawsuits against public participation (SLAPP). These SLAPP lawsuits are intended to squelch any criticism of a particular stem cell company or of physicians offering experimental stem cell procedures that might be dangerous to patients.

Even the threat of SLAPP can be powerful. For example, the ISSCR, which had taken a proactive stance on stem cell tourism a few years ago, was reportedly threatened with litigation by stem cell clinics. As a result, it has shut down its anti-stem cell tourism web portal, which had allowed concerned citizens to mention specific clinics that raised concerns.[xxii] Even so, other forms of patient advocacy persist despite threats of litigation.

For example, when University of Minnesota Professor Leigh Turner sent a public letter to the FDA raising concerns about stem cell company Celltex, both he and the University were reportedly threatened with litigation as well,[xxiii] but did not back down. To date, no lawsuit has been filed. Note that Leigh finished as the runner up in my blog's Stem Cell Person of the Year contest for 2012[xxiv] for his brave actions. I know how it feels to be in that situation as I also have been threatened with litigation in several instances, but I have maintained my position that patient safety comes first and requires action.

Interestingly, companies employing SLAPP as a strategy have to be careful, as there is an inherent danger to dubious stem cell clinics and physicians if lawsuits proceed. During the discovery phase of such cases, defendants could request and obtain substantial amounts of confidential information about the company and its practices that could open a

---

[xxii]http://www.nature.com/news/2011/110628/full/474550a.html
[xxiii]http://chronicle.com/blogs/brainstorm/celltex-says-keep-quiet-or-well-sue/44901
[xxiv]http://www.ipscell.com/2013/01/stem-cell-person-of-the-year-roman-reed/

Pandora's box for the company. This potential risk is perhaps why many stem cell companies threaten legal action, but most often do not follow through. Note that sometimes they do follow through so those of us in the advocacy community pushing for accountability in the for-profit stem cell arena are continually at real risk. Ultimately, it is organizations such as ISSCR who should be confronting dubious stem cell clinics rather than individuals. Given the growing number of non-compliant stem cell operations in the US and more globally, I believe that ISSCR must return to a more assertive stance.

The Stem Cell Black Market

Have I got a stem cell for you!

We hear a lot about the dangers of an increasing number of rogue stem cell clinics, but another critical trend has flown more under the radar: **direct marketing of stem cells to doctors.**

This is big business and arguably one of the biggest threats to patients. In some ways it is a black market right here in the US as well as more globally.

When I think of direct marketing, what pops in my heads are images of ads or little samples of products that show up in the mail.

For doctors generally, direct marketing materials might be flyers, free pill samples for patients, and so forth. However stem cell direct marketing to doctors amazingly can involve actual living stem cells that hucksters are trying, sometimes successfully, to convince doctors to inject into patients. In the same way that there is a black market for body parts,[xxv] a black market in stem cells is emerging as well (Figure 8.4).

At the stem cell meeting called the World Stem Cell Summit[xxvi] in 2012, a doctor who was giving a talk said a man showed up at his office and said he had **sample stem cells in his pocket** available to doctors at that practice for use in treating patients.

[xxv]http://www.nytimes.com/2012/06/29/world/europe/black-market-for-body-parts-spreads-in-europe.html?pagewanted=all&_r=0
[xxvi]http://www.worldstemcellsummit.com

This reminds me of the stereotypic huckster on the street corner in New York City who lifts up his sleeve, which is ringed with a dozen watches, or opens his trench coat and says with a grin "wanna buy a watch?" except in this case if even a few doctors buy the "black market" stem cells, patients will be put at serious risk beyond a faulty watch.

What are these supposed "stem cells"?

According to experts, they can be almost anything including some disturbing possibilities.

Sheep cells are popular. Other black market stem cells might be human amniotic, placental, or umbilical cord cells obtained without consent from mothers at the maternity wing of a hospital, essentially stolen by someone who works there.

Could these "vendors" be licensed to sell stem cells? Given the surreptitious nature of the transactions involved, this seems very unlikely.

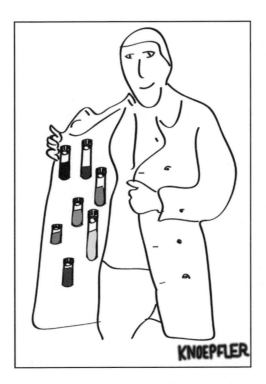

Figure 8.4. My View of A Stem Cell Black Marketeer.

Another dangerous form of direct marketing in the stem cell field that is exploding right now is of **kits for supposed stem cell purification**. Such a kit allows a doctor to, for example, take a blob of fat and allegedly turn it into purified fat stem cells. This is big business, mainly for preparation of stem cells for autologous transplants, according to several stem cell doctors that I have talked to recently in this arena.

The dangers in such kits include that they enable inexperienced doctors to offer procedures that they are not trained or qualified to perform, and that such kits may not actually work properly or may change stem cells in ways that make them drugs. It is also difficult for the FDA to oversee such kits if they are direct-marketed to physicians.

It is some physicians in the for-profit stem cell field who have informed me about these kits and the dangers they see of the kits promoting unsafe stem cell interventions by doctors who are newbies to the stem cell world.

Much the same as the issue of fake patients, the stem cell black market is a key dangerous development, but one that has not received sufficient attention.

Non-Compliant Predictions

Increased patient lawsuits against non-compliant stem cell doctors and clinics

I believe that a growing trend in the future, perhaps already emerging today, will be patients suing providers of stem cell interventions for fraud or malpractice (if the providers even were doctors). Of course while being sued is not an indication of guilt, the increasing number of non-compliant stem cell providers operating around the world and their increasing customer base will lead to more lawsuits.

We do not yet know the outcome of the litigation surrounding the fraud allegations against RNL Bio mentioned earlier and they could be found innocent, but an earlier case that has gone into the law books is informative. For better or worse, I called it the "Stem Cell Supermodel Case" on my blog.[xxvii]

[xxvii]http://www.ipscell.com/2012/07/testimony-in-shocking-supermodel-stem-cell-fraud-case-i-lied-to-patients/

"I lied to patients," testified a weeping, young woman in court.

She had worked as an office assistant at a company that injected bogus and potentially dangerous cow-based "stem cell" products into human patients. This company, which in different incarnations went by various names including Biomark in the US, was at the center of a dramatic global case of alleged stem cell fraud and criminal misconduct.[xxviii]

The Biomark case swept across the globe including the US, the Netherlands, and South Africa. Importantly the two defendants in the Biomark case were Americans, Stephen van Rooyen and his "supermodel" wife, Laura Brown. The plaintiff was one Justine Asher. She sued van Rooyen and Brown, who ran the company called Biomark International in the US until it was shut down in 2003 related to alleged criminal activity.

Prior to treating Asher in the Netherlands, van Rooyen and Brown had several years earlier reportedly[xxix] fled the US as fugitives to escape a federal criminal indictment[xxx] listing dozens of charges for their actions at Biomark. Reportedly for a time they were on the FBI's most wanted list.

Brown at some point adopted the alias "Sean Castle" and Van Rooyen became "Sebastian Carlisle" according to court testimony. It is unclear why they chose those names, but both had the same S.C. initials that could also stand for "Stem Cell". The US reportedly was working to have Brown and van Rooyen extradited back to the US as recently as 2011. As of the press time of this book I could not determine if the extradition case was still pending.

Asher, who likely was unaware of Brown and van Rooyen's earlier alleged criminal conduct in the US related to stem cell procedures, was given a "stem cell" transplant in the Netherlands around 2006. van Rooyen and Brown allegedly told Asher that the procedure would make

---

[xxviii]http://www.iol.co.za/news/south-africa/i-lied-to-patients-says-distraught-woman-1.674030#.UAX6XI6bGPB
[xxix]http://www.iol.co.za/news/south-africa/paraplegic-gets-nod-to-sue-stem-cell-pair-1.303873#.UVC_cY6bFVS
[xxx]http://www.circare.org/lex/06cr1534_indictment.pdf

Asher miraculously walk again. Ms. Asher is a paraplegic due to injuries suffered in a car accident that broke her neck.

The procedure that Asher received sounds very dangerous. It was reportedly a "cocktail" that included bovine cells grown in fetal bovine serum that was injected into her neck and IV into her arm.

Muddying the waters, the new company in the Netherlands that van Rooyen and Brown opened up at which Asher apparently got her procedure was called Advanced Cell Therapeutics (ACT), not to be confused with the current, legit stem cell company headquartered in the US going by the same acronym, Advanced Cell Technology (ACT), which is now conducting several early stage clinical trials based on embryonic stem cells as discussed earlier.

The woman who testified that she inadvertently lied to patients while working as a personal assistant for Brown and van Rooyen at Biomark was one Danielle Jibrail. She also testified that Biomark became the "new" company called Advanced Cell Therapeutics specifically for the purpose of avoiding negative reports about Biomark in the press. Reportedly Brown and van Rooyen also gave many (more than 50 in the US alone) patients "stem cell procedures" for MS and ALS.[xxxi]

According to her testimony, Jibrail came to discover later that van Rooyen and Brown gave patients potentially dangerous procedures and collected large sums of money from the patients, while they lived an "extravagant lifestyle":

> Jibrail told the court she later spoke to a doctor who worked for ACT, Catherine Orridge, who told her the stem cells came from California, and were meant for research purposes. They were not fit for humans. Jibrail said she logged on to the Internet and looked into the matter.
>
> "Then I knew that Laura or Steve did not care about the patients they were treating," she said, becoming emotional.

[xxxi]http://io9.com/5651791/doctor-injected-ms-and-als-patients-with-bovine-stem-cells-as-part-of-fraudulent-cure-medical-panel-says

"They lived very extravagant lifestyles and spent the money patients paid them on entertainment."

After that Jibrail contacted the FBI and emailed patients the "truth", before later resigning. Getting back to the patient Asher who sued, reportedly she won her case.[xxxii] As a result, van Rooyen and Brown had to sell their mansion in 2011 to pay the damages. Adding further intrigue to the case, Brown reportedly died under mysterious circumstances shortly thereafter in Cape Town in 2011.[xxxiii] The extradition lawyer website reporting the death said:

"Brown, who had been separated from Van Rooyen, is said to have been suffering from depression since she lost their plush mansion due to financial problems."

To my knowledge to date the cause of death for Brown remains unknown or at least not publicly available. One can see from this case how some companies seeking to profit from dubious stem cell procedures put patients at risk. The people running such companies adopt many strategies including moving around the globe, secrecy, changing their names and their company names, and outright deception to make profits. However, in the end such efforts ultimately do not keep them out of trouble. I think such companies will face an increasing onslaught of litigation from patients.

A Deregulated Stem Cell Future?

What will the future be like if the proponents of full stem cell deregulation win out? In the cartoon in Figure 8.5, I imagine a world in which stem cell deregulation has gone to an extreme where patients can receive stem cell injections via a drive-thru like a burger or a cup of coffee.

[xxxii]http://www.legalbrief.co.za/article.php?story=20110308131840325
[xxxiii]http://internationalextraditionblog.com/tag/steve-van-rooyen-and-laura-brown/

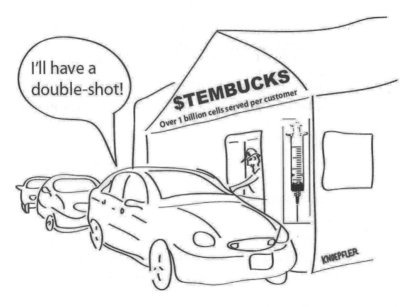

Figure 8.5. An envisioned deregulated stem cell future where patients can get transplants of stem cells in a drive-thru setting.

While I do not envisage the particularly extreme future depicted in the cartoon becoming reality, the point is that the greater extent that one deregulates stem cells the higher the risk to patients. Some advocates of stem cell deregulation have a conflict of interest because they want to make more money at the expense of patient safety.

Summary

The goal for the stem cell field is to have our innovation and ethics too. I believe it is not just desirable, but also possible to do both. A number of stem cell for-profits have demonstrated the ability to maintain creative, productive, and ethical operations. As a realist, I understand that others will choose money over ethics, putting patients at risk of injury or death in the process. It is the responsibility of the stem cell field to promote ethical applications. We should identify and reward ethical innovators, but also collectively hold those putting patients at risk accountable ideally through action by societies such as ISSCR.

References

1. Amariglio, N, et al. (2009) Donor-derived brain tumor following neural stem cell transplantation in an ataxia telangiectasia patient. *PLoS medicine.* **6**:2:e1000029.
2. Knoepfler, PS (2013) Call for fellowship programs in stem cell-based regenerative and cellular medicine: new stem cell training is essential for physicians. *Regenerative medicine.* **8**:2:223-5.
3. Mitka, M (2010) Troubled by "stem cell tourism" claims, group launches web-based guidance. *JAMA: the journal of the American Medical Association.* **304**:12:1315-6.
4. Caulfield, TA Zarzeczny (2012) Stem cell tourism and Canadian family physicians. *Canadian family physician Medecin de famille canadien.* **58**:4:365-8, e182-5.
5. Sleeboom-Faulkner, MPK Patra (2011) Experimental stem cell therapy: biohierarchies and bionetworking in Japan and India. *Social studies of science.* **41**:5:645-66.
6. Jawad, S, et al. (2012) Safeguarding patients against stem cell tourism. *The British journal of general practice: the journal of the Royal College of General Practitioners.* **62**:598:269-70.

Chapter 9

Patient Bill of Rights and Guide to Stem Cell Treatments

Patients are an ever growing, valuable and very welcome part of the stem cell community. Since starting my blog more than two years ago, I have had the good fortune to meet many patients and patient advocates interested in stem cell-based therapies. They provide much needed context for understanding how best to make safe and effective stem cell procedures a reality.

As a cancer patient myself I can relate to what patients who have received life-changing medical diagnoses are going through and the urgency they feel. I know why some are considering stem cell procedures because I understand the importance of hope. In this chapter I guide you through the key factors in the world of stem cell procedures, provide a novel Stem Cell Patient Bill of Rights, and list my concerns about non-compliant treatments. **Note that this chapter is not intended as medical advice.**

Advocacy

Stem cell patient advocates are patients or those advocating for them who have the passion to change the stem cell world. They often work to pass legislation to support research or other efforts they see as beneficial to patients. Advocates also sometimes are active in promoting research and fund-raising for specific institutions or scientists. Patient advocates play powerful roles in many capacities such as via sitting on FDA panels and serving on grant funding agency boards (e.g. CIRM). They also conduct outreach to educate other patients, political leaders, and the general public on diseases and potential stem cell therapies.

The outreach efforts of patients and advocates are also targeted to scientists to bring the all-important patient perspective to research. One of the great challenges to advancing stem cell-based medicines is the invisible wall between patients and scientists. As both a scientist and a cancer patient I see it as my job to break down this wall. I have had some success in recent years in bringing different parties together through bridge building. However, sadly most stem cell scientists remain largely inaccessible to patients because the scientists mistakenly believe that there should be a distance, a wall between them and patients.

Attributes of successful patient advocates

Patient advocates are heroes and achieve remarkable things. They have a knack for breaking down walls between patients and scientists! Some advocates go above and beyond the call of duty to be model advocates and I want to commend them for their leadership here.

Roman Reed is one of the model advocates. He won my blog's Stem Cell 2012 Person of the Year Award for many reasons[i] (e.g. he and his foundation[ii] do amazing things). He is the complete package of a patient advocate.

How so?

There is a reason Roman is a mentor and role model to so many other patient advocates, who can learn from Roman's example in some key areas:

- He does his homework and knows the science (see us talking about some unpublished preclinical data from my lab in Figure 9.1).
- He focuses on the positive rather than the negative.
- He makes real, tangible things happen such as laws.
- He knows the importance of funding as the fuel for making stem cell medicine a reality.

---

[i]http://www.ipscell.com/2013/01/stem-cell-person-of-the-year-roman-reed/
[ii]http://romanreedfoundation.com/

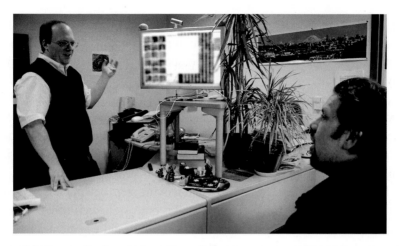

Figure 9.1. Roman Reed and the author talking over some preclinical data from the Knoepfler lab in 2013.

- He is a uniter and not a divider, building bridges between all kinds of folks who might normally be separated: scientists, advocates, politicians, lawyers, patients, funding agency folks, etc.
- He empowers others rather than working to consolidate power for himself.

I consider myself sort of a newbie patient advocate being active in the area just for a few years and I find myself learning from Roman all the time. I wish Roman would teach a class on patient advocacy. He has mentored many other leading stem cell and spinal cord injury (SCI) patient advocates.

There are more outstanding patient advocates as well and one is Roman's father, **Don C. Reed**, who has been instrumental in key positive developments in the field including making CIRM a reality. There are others who make a powerful difference (listed below alphabetically by first name).

Bernard (Bernie) Siegel is the head of Genetics Policy Institute.[iii] Bernie is also the organizer of the annual World Stem Cell Summit[iv] (more on that later in the Chapter), a very patient-friendly meeting. He is

---

[iii]http://www.genpol.org/
[iv]http://www.worldstemcellsummit.com/

the tireless engine that drives stem cell advocacy and accountability. It is hard to imagine the stem cell community today without Bernie's contributions over the years. Bernie empowers and educates in a global way like no other.

Judy Roberson is a stem cell advocate for Huntington's Disease (HD) who has made great strides in education about this important disease. She also has been a driving force for obtaining substantial research funding for doing research on using stem cells to treat HD. In this radio interview you can listen and learn from Judy.[v]

Katie Sharify is a very effective and moving stem cell patient advocate. Katie is a participant in the Geron embryonic stem cell-based clinical trial for SCI (now going to be run by BioTime) and a patient advocate. Katie is that rare person who has the courage to tell her story and inspire others. One way she does this is through YouTube and other Videos.[vi,vii]

Sabrina Cohen is a long-time stem cell and (SCI) research patient advocate. She is the founder of the Sabrina Cohen Foundation,[viii] which does great things such as raising awareness through lecture series and funding of research. Sabrina is a high-profile advocate who extends our community's messages to an incredibly important, larger audience. She is a moving and powerful speaker. She received the prestigious Inspiration Award at the 2012 World Stem Cell Summit meeting.[ix]

Ted Harada, a patient advocate for amyotrophic lateral sclerosis (ALS), makes a huge, tangible difference. Ted is very active in promoting safe and effective stem cell treatments as well as working to get these therapies to the patients who might benefit from them. He was one of the first patients in NeuralStem's ALS clinical trial and had a striking response to the therapy. Ted was nominated for my lab's Stem Cell Person of the Year Award and his nominator said of Ted, "He became a vocal advocate for stem cell trials in ALS community." You can read more about Ted here on CNN Health.[x]

---

[v]http://www.blogtalkradio.com/help4hd/2012/01/23/the-hd-view-with-judy-roberson
[vi]http://www.youtube.com/watch?v=zX1vHnXlvgs
[vii]http://www.youtube.com/watch?v=kqEZ4faoVpU
[viii]http://sabrinacohenfoundation.org/
[ix]http://cirmresearch.blogspot.com/2012/12/sabrina-cohen-honored-for-providing.html
[x]http://www.cnn.com/2011/09/28/health/early-als-trial-results-encouraging/index.html

TJ Atchison. The person who nominated TJ for my lab's Stem Cell Person of the Year 2012 award said, "TJ is an inspiration and hero". TJ suffered a SCI and became the first ever embryonic stem cell-based clinical trial participant. He worked to make The TJ Atchison Spinal Cord Injury Research Program[xi] a reality via the TJ Atchison SCI Research Act. His nominator also said, "The impact of this new effort will be tremendous".

Of course this list of great patient advocates is not all inclusive and there are many others who make major positive impacts.

Stem Cell Patient's Bill of Rights

I believe that patients seeking out stem cell procedures should have specific rights. I outline and discuss these in my Stem Cell Patient's Bill of Rights (Figure 9.2).

Stem Cell Patient Bill of Rights

Article One, The Right to Truly Informed Consent.

Article Two, The Right to Treatment by a Trained Provider.

Article Three, The Right to Have Your Stem Cells Be Prepared in a GMP Facility.

Article Four, The Right to Continuing Follow Up by the Provider.

Article Five, The Right to Ownership of Your Stem Cells.

Article Six, The Right to Expanded Compassionate Use For Fatal Diseases.

Article Seven, The Right to be in a Clinical Trial for Experimental Procedures.

Article Eight, The Right to Not to be Charged for Clinical Trial Participation.

Article Nine, The Right to Full Disclosure of Anticipated Costs.

Active Ten, The Right to be Treated Regardless of Socioeconomic Status.

Paul Knoepfler

Figure 9.2. A Stem Cell Patient Bill of Rights, containing ten articles (rights) that patients should have when getting a stem cell procedure.

[xi]http://www.uab.edu/medicine/tjatchisonprogram/

Article one: The right to truly informed consent

As a stem cell patient you should have the right to be properly informed by your medical provider of the potential risks and benefits of the procedure you are contemplating before you consent. How can you give your informed consent as a patient if the medical provider lies by omission by not telling you pertinent information about risks or if they claim safety when there is no data? How can you as a patient give informed consent if the provider makes claims of efficacy that are not based on evidence, but rather anecdote? The answer is that you cannot. The patient should also be made aware if the stem cell procedure is not FDA approved. As a patient you have the right to be informed.

Before you or a loved one gets a stem cell treatment, you also have the right to see the actual data that relate to the procedure's safety and efficacy. See what kind of answer you get when you ask a provider to go over the data with them. If they criticize the FDA then that is a warning flag. If they refuse to show you data, then that is also a big red warning flag. They may say the data is confidential or that it is not published yet or that you are not knowledge enough to understand it. Do not accept these excuses. As a patient I believe that you have a right to see the data, assuming they have any data at all, and have your doctor explain it to you.

In addition, patients should be informed by providers of any potential conflicts of interest (COIs). For example, if the doctor is an owner or investor in a company or companies with intellectual property rights to the technology being used, the patient should be informed of that COI. If the company is publicly traded, the patient should be made aware if their provider owns stock in the company as that is a COI as well.

Article two: The right to receive treatment by a trained provider

Stem cell patients have the right to be treated by a provider who is educated and trained in stem cell biology, transplantation, regulatory and ethical issues. See my proposed physician fellowship curriculum (Figure 8.2) in the previous chapter.

Article three: The right to have your stem cells be prepared in a GMP facility

Stem cell patients should have the right to have their stem cells, if they are processed or grown in a lab, to be handled in a GMP (Good Manufacturing Practices) or equivalent facility. Patients should not have to wonder if their stem cells are contaminated by shoddy practices.

Article four: The right to continuing follow up by the provider

Patients have the right to proper medical follow up by the provider who gave them the stem cell procedure and that follow up should last years, if not decades. Follow up is important for patient safety and for obtaining information about the safety and efficacy of stem cell procedures.

Article five: The right to ownership of your stem cells

I believe that patients have the right to ownership of their stem cells unless they make the conscious decision to give up that right. As discussed in the next chapter that right is not the default situation today in many cases. Patients have be assertive and very careful about what they sign to retain the rights to their own stem cells. While access to patient samples is essential for progress in research and biorepositories are critical tools for clinical research, patients should not automatically give up all of their rights to their own cells or products derived from them. Physicians should talk with patients about rights such as to their own tissues and cells, but it is somewhat of a taboo topic.

Article six: The right to expanded compassionate use for fatal diseases under appropriate conditions

Patients facing terminal illnesses such as ALS for which there is no other effective treatment should have greater access to compassionate use of stem cell therapies. Careful expansion of compassionate use of stem cells is something I favor as I mentioned earlier, but it must be subject to very clear rules and be coupled to thorough informed consent. We do not want to create an out-of-control, even dangerous situation for thousands of patients as we have seen recently in 2013 in Italy (see the previous chapter), which has overly permissive rules for compassionate use of stem cells. What would be most helpful to patients overall is a balanced approach to compassionate use, neither too permissive nor too restrictive.

Article seven: The right to be in a clinical trial for experimental procedures

Patients who are given experiment stem cell procedures have the right to be part of a clinical trial. Outside of that context, vulnerable patients can be taken advantage of and are exposed to much greater risks.

Article eight: The right to not be charged for clinical trial participation

I believe that patients should be able to participate in clinical trials without being charged. Unfortunately today some dubious clinics charge patients up to tens of thousands of dollars to receive stem cell procedures that are technically part of clinical trials.

Article nine: The right to full disclosure of anticipated costs

Patients who get stem cell treatments sometimes tell me that after getting one treatment that the clinics only then recommend additional treatments. In fact the patients are often told only after the fact of the first treatment that repeated treatments give them the best chance of positive results. As a patient you should have the right to know the predicted total cost that you will incur for a full-spectrum of treatments that are given to the average patient at that clinic. For example, if the average customer at that clinic receives three twenty thousand dollar treatments, new potential customers should be told that the anticipated cost might be $60,000 not $20,000.

Article ten: The right to be treated regardless of socioeconomic status

People should have the opportunity to receive stem cell treatments regardless of their socioeconomic status. This issue will become increasingly important as new, expensive stem cell treatments are approved in the coming decade. The best stem cell-based medicine should not be available only to the rich. It certainly is not clear how many stem cell treatments will be covered by The Affordable Care Act here in the US, but many surely will not.

An Insider's Guide to Stem Cell Procedures

It is very difficult for patients to know what they are getting themselves or their loved ones into when they buy a stem cell procedure from a for-profit clinic, especially if that clinic is unlicensed or out of the country. Even in the US, however, the water is very muddy when it comes to getting solid information on non-compliant stem cell clinics.

Here I provide a guide to evaluating stem cell clinics and potential procedures. My intention with this guide is not to substitute for your working with your physician to decide what to do or not to do, but rather to provide an overall framework for thinking about stem cell procedures including their potential benefits and the many, complex risks. **This guide is not intended as medical advice.**

My main focus in this guide is on procedures offered by for-profit clinics operating in an unlicensed manner, but some of this advice could also prove useful in a broader sense such as when considering whether to participate in a clinical trial on stem cells, perhaps even at a big academic teaching hospital or university.

Ten things to consider before getting a stem cell procedure for yourself or a loved one

I know there are thousands of people out there looking for more practical information about stem cell therapies and procedures. These folks understandably are using the Internet to look for some clear, reliable info on stem cell procedures either for themselves or their loved ones. Too often the material that is out there is wrong, misleading, based on conflicts of interest, or overly complex.

I want to address this need for information speaking as a scientist, patient advocate and cancer survivor in the form of 10 key facts to help you and your family to guide your way through the jungle of information and noise out there about stem cells.

Number one: Lab-produced stem cells are a drug and possibly permanent once in your body

In my opinion (and that of the FDA as well as federal courts to date), **lab-produced stem cells are drugs**. Yes, they are very unusual drugs, but they are drugs. Unlike other drugs, once a patient receives a stem cell drug, it will not necessarily simply go away because a stem cell drug consists of living cells that often behave in unpredictable ways. What this means is that if the stem cells are doing bad things then your doctor has no way to stop it. By contrast if you take aspirin or blood-pressure medication or some other traditional pill-based drug, if you have a bad reaction, you can stop taking the pill and your body eliminates the drug within a period of days. There may still be longer-term side effects, but the cause is gone. In contrast, stem cells, should they cause a negative reaction, cannot be removed.

Number two: There will be side effects

Like any medical product, even aspirin, **stem cells procedures will have side effects**. Not "maybe". Definitely. The hope is the side effects will be relatively mild. Any doctor or clinic that tells potential patients that the stem cells proposed to be used for a procedure will not have side effects is failing in their duty to the patient.

If you receive a stem cell transplant, your body will react to it and have side effects of some kind. The question is how mild or severe will the reaction to the stem cells be? The hope is that in many cases the side effects will be so mild that you are not even aware of them, but it is difficult to predict what will happen for any one specific patient.

Number three: Most stem cell procedures sold in the US are not approved by the FDA

The FDA has not approved stem cell treatments except bone marrow transplant/hematopoietic stem cell transplantation. What this means is that other stem cell procedures that you see advertised on the Internet that indicate they will be given to you inside the US have a much higher risk of being unsafe. The exception to this is if a procedure is part of an FDA-approved clinical trial. Outside of that domain, stem cell procedures most often have not been carefully evaluated prior to their use in patients. It is important to note as well that even FDA-approved clinical trials can have substantial risks.

Number four: Outside the US use extra caution with stem cell procedures

We have to avoid the ethnocentric trap of thinking that only the US can offer advanced medical procedures such as those based on stem cells, but on the other hand within the US at least you have the added safety of the FDA, which provides some measure, albeit imperfect, of protection. In the vast majority of other countries regulatory agencies are practically non-existent or are far less strict than the FDA. Nonetheless, a large number of patients travel to other countries for experimental stem cell procedures (a phenomenon called "stem cell tourism"). The risks with such procedures are unclear, but probably very high.

Number five: Stem cells are not a cure all

I am as excited as anybody about the potential of stem cells to treat a wide variety of diseases and injuries, but stem cells are not a miracle cure for everything. When a doctor offers to inject some kind of stem cells or a stem cell-derived product into a patient either into the bloodstream or a specific place that is injured such as a shoulder, we just do not know at this point if it will do any good with the exception of bone marrow transplant.

If the doctor, clinic staff, or supposed patients who have already received an experimental therapy from the clinic talk about "cures" or use other over-the-top language, consider that a red flag. Another indication of trouble is if the clinic has a long laundry list of diseases that it claims its stem cell products can treat or cure. As a stem cell scientist, I am ready to admit that stem cells are no panacea so when you see that broad, pie-in-the-sky claim, you can bet the people making it either know very little about stem cells or are engaging in false advertising (or both).

Number six: Do not let celebrities guide your medical decisions

The number of famous people getting stem cell procedures is increasing including sports stars and celebrities. My advice is to not let what these celebs do influence what you decide to do about your health. Just because they are famous, do not believe for one minute that they are any more informed than you or your personal doctor about medical procedures or stem cells. If anything I think sometimes famous people are more reckless with their health than average people like you and me. In addition, after reading this book you certainly know more than the typical celebrity about stem cells.

Number seven: Reach out to scientists for dialogue

As a scientist I am always happy to hear from people outside the scientific community who have questions about stem cells and other research. We should not offer medical advice (I never do), but we can give our perspectives on stem cell research and its clinical potential. I would advise that you do not cold call scientists on the phone as you are unlikely to reach them that way. Instead consider the option of emailing. I cannot speak for all stem cell scientists but you might be surprised at how likely it is that if you send them a very short, clear email with one or two polite questions that they will respond and be helpful. You can often find scientists' emails on the Internet or in their published papers, some of which are usually publicly available.

Number eight: The people selling you non-FDA approved stem cell procedures want your money

Most of the people out there advertising stem cell procedures that are not FDA approved are only really after one thing: your money. As such they will do their best to convince you that their procedure is safe and effective. They may offer testimonials either from patients who truly believe they were helped or from people who play patients on the Internet. The bottom line is that the sellers of dubious stem cell procedures simply want your money. If they were truly some kind of Robin Hoods of medicine or heroes wouldn't they be offering stem cell procedures for free or at least not for incredibly high fees such as tens of thousands of dollars?

Number nine: There is no such thing as completely "proven safe"

Patients or their families contact me regularly. They often mention that the doctors offering stem cell procedures told them that the procedures are proven safe and that your own stem cells cannot harm you or that adult stem cells are harmless. You should be skeptical if you hear such claims. A responsible physician and clinic will discuss risks with you, not claim there are no risks.

Number ten: Be wary of patient testimonials

Patient testimonials are a very powerful marketing tool used by non-compliant stem cell clinics. It is standard practice for the websites of such businesses to have videos of patients stating that the procedures being sold worked for them and had no side effects. Such claims, if made instead directly by the company itself, are open to scrutiny and even legal action by the FDA. However, when claims are made by patients, even on a company's website, they are more difficult to deal with by regulators. In essence, businesses put patient testimonials up on their websites because they work to draw in new patients and boost cash flow, but at the same time it allows for claims to be made about the procedures without the company risking to do that themselves. Even so many companies themselves do make many claims not based on evidence.

Eight simple reasons to think twice before getting an unlicensed stem cell procedure today

If you do a Google search for the key phrase "stem cell treatment", in your search results you will get dozens of hits that include clinics all over the world offering stem cell procedures including in the US. In the list below, I go step by step through eight key reasons why I do not recommend that patients get unlicensed stem cell procedures from non-compliant clinics today.

Reason 1: Lack of patient follow-up

An integral part of FDA-sanctioned clinical trials is follow-up, which means the clinical trial follows patients in the long term to see how they are doing and monitor for adverse outcomes that can then be logged and treated. A challenge for a clinic trial is patients who, for whatever reason not integral to the trial, are lost to follow-up, which means that the doctor and clinic completely lose track of a given patient forever. Patients are sometimes lost to follow up in even the best clinical trials. However, some stem cell clinics' way of doing business almost guarantees that many if not most of their patients are lost to follow-up.

The vast majority of non-compliant for-profit, point-of-care stem cell clinics do not do any significant follow-up unless it is to work to convince the patients to get more procedures. A lack of follow-up is problematic for many reasons. First of all, it means we all learn less about the potential strengths and weaknesses of new stem cell therapies. It also puts patients at greater risk for serious treatment-related health problems, which when they occur are liable to remain untreated for a longer period of time absent follow up.

Why would clinics choose not to do follow-up? Follow-up is labor intensive and costly. Imagine if you treat 100 patients with stem cells, collect the payments, and send them on their way (maybe you have one post-procedure visit with the patient) versus following the patients for say 10 years with regular appointments (low profit-margin activities). The former is not scientifically or medically the proper thing to do, but it sure is dramatically cheaper than the latter. However, the latter provides more data and protects patients.

Reason 2: Possible exclusion from future clinical trials

By getting an unlicensed stem cell procedure patients may be excluded from participation in a clinical trial in the future. By receiving an unlicensed treatment, without realizing it most of the time (I believe) patients are in essence putting a big black check mark on any future clinical trial participation pre-screening form, perhaps leading to their exclusion. Why? Because by their nature unlicensed stem cell procedures are nebulous and could confound a given patient's results in a future trial.

This could be disastrous. We will take a hypothetical patient as an example who has a back injury and receives an unlicensed stem cell procedure consisting of an injection of stem cells (or more often multiple injections). A few years later an FDA-approved clinical trial begins for treating back injury using stem cells and this trial seems very promising based on extensive, encouraging pre-clinical data. Our hypothetical patient may not be able to participate in this new trial. As a result they may have in essence harmed themselves and been harmed by the doctor doing the earlier unlicensed stem cell therapy since it led to their exclusion from the future clinical trial.

When I have had discussions about this issue with patients who advocate unlicensed stem cell procedures some say, "who will know?" and "what would simply stop me from not mentioning my previous unlicensed treatment?" I suppose this is true, but in that case you are actually harming science, medicine, and possibly other patients because your previous unlicensed procedure may screw up the results of the new clinical trial.

Reason 3: Undesired, non-cancerous tissue growth

One dangerous issue seems to fly under the radar of most patients getting unlicensed stem cell procedures: undesired tissue growth.

So what are stem cells again? They are potent cells that can differentiate into a number of cell types and they also self-renew. What this means is that the stem cells can make multiple other types of differentiated cells or more of themselves. Focusing on the former quality, even adult stem cells such as the ever-touted adipose-derived MSCs can express multiple personalities when they differentiate. They can form more of themselves, but also they can make fat, bone, cartilage, blood vessels, and other cell types.

That is good right?

Well, yes and no.

It is good if you want to make a variety of cell types, but it is bad in the sense that MSCs are being used by unlicensed clinics in very "blunt" ways. An example of this is the "stem cell face lift" in which fat MSCs are injected into the face. If they just make a bit of subcutaneous fat then in theory they could "smooth out" wrinkles, but what if these MSCs decide for whatever reason they will become an undesired tissue type in your face?

For example, what if in your cheek a piece of cartilage or a rapidly-growing mass of bone forms? What if the MSCs sprout a mass of blood vessels all over your face? Dr. Allan Wu presented the now famous case at the 2012 World Stem Cell Summit of the woman who had received dangerous stem cell facelift conducted by another physician. After the experimental procedure, the woman fairly quickly developed a serious, but puzzling eye problem and turned to Dr. Wu for help.

Dr. Wu investigated and determined that most likely the injected MSCs for the face-lift by the other doctor had grown bone in the skin next to her eye, bone that grew onto existing tissue and could have blinded this woman. This is serious. One cannot just assume that adipose-derived MSCs will do only one thing especially in the context of procedure administered by a non-compliant clinic and untrained doctor.

Reason 4: Cancerous growth from transplanted stem cells

Unfortunately even normal stem cells are cellular relatives to cancer cells. There is no getting around this relationship. While various techniques are used in some cases to lower the risk of stem cells causing cancer in patients (e.g. pre-differentiation of the stem cells into cells of specific types that will not grow as we discussed earlier in the book), there is always going to be some risk of transplanted stem cells growing a malignant tumor in the patient. The goal is to make that risk as close to zero as possible.

Reason 5: Autoimmune problems

Stem cells do not have to grow to cause problems. When stem cells are transplanted from one part of the body to another or from one patient to another, the immune system may be activated leading to disease. Many patients seeking stem cell procedures already have an autoimmune disease such as Multiple Sclerosis, heightening the risk of a stem cell-based immune reaction.

Reason 6: Jeopardizing ownership of your own cells

When I talk with patients who advocate for less regulatory oversight of stem cell therapies one common refrain I hear is, "my cells belong to me, they are not a drug, and no one should be able to tell me what I can or cannot do with them including the FDA."

I am a proponent of the concept that patients should have rights to cells isolated or produced from them as mentioned in my Stem Cell Patient Bill of Rights earlier in this chapter.

Unfortunately, however, the notion that we each own our cells even once they are removed from our bodies is on shaky legal ground at best. In fact, the current legal precedents would suggest that once separated from our bodies, even under false pretenses, the more probable default outcome is that we have few legal rights to those cells (unless we are talking about embryos made by IVF). There are some state laws that might help patients reserve rights to their tissues, but only rarely.

In general, if patients want to have the best chance of retaining rights to their cells they must be proactive, educate themselves, be largely unwilling to blindly sign just any release forms given to them by doctors or clinics, and be quite assertive.

In the stem cell field specifically, the same concerns apply. In many cases patients who assume they own their stem cells removed from their bodies, particularly if the stem cells have been grown in culture (making them distinct from the patient's endogenous stem cells), may be mistaken. It all depends on the fine print in that consent/release form you signed as a patient.

To my knowledge, there is no clear court precedent supporting stem cell ownership by patients. However, to the contrary, several legal and historical cases suggest quite the opposite. A reading of them helps provide context for how physicians and courts would be liable to handle the issue of cell ownership should a conflict arise in the near future, which I predict is quite likely.

In the now well known case of Henrietta Lacks, so eloquently described by writer Rebecca Skloot in her book *The Immortal Life of Henrietta Lacks [1]*, we learn that Ms. Lacks was betrayed by her own doctor who secretly grew cells from a cancer that had stricken Ms. Lacks. He established what is called an immortal cell line called HeLa from the cancer. Generally most cells taken from patients are mortal and will stop growing and die or senesce after a relatively short period of time in the lab. In contrast, some cancers such as Ms. Lacks' contain cells that can, under the right conditions or with certain manipulations, live forever. Somewhere during the cancer formation process cells became immortalized. Such cells can be useful tools for research and lucrative products. Ms. Lacks and her family never consented for her cancer to be used in this way and never received any compensation.

Another cancer patient's situation led to an influential, although puzzling court decision related to cell ownership. A man named John Moore had the misfortune of having an unusual kind of blood cancer called "hairy cell leukemia". Physician Dr. David W. Golde treated Moore.

During the course of following up on treatment, Dr. Golde apparently realized that Moore's cells may be very useful for biomedical science and in fact could be commercialized. During the years after Moore's diagnosis and treatment, on a regular basis Golde took biological samples from Moore. The isolation of the samples for a time had

Moore's consent, but Golde reportedly did not inform Moore of his intent to commercialize a product from Moore's cells.

At some point, when Moore was asked to sign additional release and consent forms, it dawned on him that he might be being exploited. Golde, an employee of the University of California (UC) System (disclosure, I am an employee of the UC System), filed a patent together with the UC system for the product (the so-called "Mo" immortal cell line) derived from Moore's cells.

Ultimately, Moore sued Gold and the UC Regents after becoming aware of the commercialization of his cells without his informed consent [2].[xii] Remarkably, the California Supreme Court ruled in the *Moore v. Regents of the University of California* case that Moore could not claim a property right to his cells, but without a logical reason. The Court indicated that the highest priority was to protect the beneficial role of patient samples in biomedical research, which took precedent over an individual's rights to his cells.

The Court also ruled that the doctor had had a duty (at which he failed) to inform Moore that the doctors might make a profit off of the cells. The most important point, however, for our discussion is that Moore did not have any rights to his own cells according to the Court.

Other court rulings have supported that conclusion.

In the decision in the case of *Greenberg v. Miami Childrens Research* involving an illness called Canavan Disease,[xiii] the ruling of a US District Court was that patients do not own their cellular/tissue specimens after researchers take them for testing.[xiv]

In the case of *Catalano v. Washington University*, the university sought successfully to establish the claim of ownership of a prostate

---

[xii]From *Contested Cells* "...Moore was under the impression that all of the doctors' actions were medically indicated, and therefore he did not consider that he consented to any additional procedures which contributed directly to the eventual commercial exploitation of his cells by Golde. It was only after he was asked to waive any rights that he or his heirs may have with respect to the cell line developed from his bone marrow that he became suspicious."
[xiii]http://ghr.nlm.nih.gov/condition/canavan-disease
[xiv]http://en.wikipedia.org/wiki/Greenberg_v._Miami_Children's_Hospital_Research_Institute

cancer biorepository (a bank of tissue specimens). In a thoughtful article on this case [3], it is pointed out how both patients and institutions may rightfully want a say in the fate of biological specimens, but the author Lynn Dressler rightly argues that respect for patients is crucial:

> "It is not difficult to understand the desire of Washington University to protect its interests in a biorepository it maintained, administered, funded, and staffed and for which it assumed the legal, regulatory, and compliance risks. Nor it is surprising, given the facts of the case and legal precedence about "human specimens as property", that the Court would decide that Washington University is "the true and rightful owner and possessor of all biological materials including but not limited to blood, tissue and DNA samples...". It is disheartening, however, that the Court chose to frame the issues involved as a narrow problem of ownership at the expense of appreciating the importance of maintaining a respectful and trusting relationship with current and potential research participants."

Dressler also nicely frames the key point in her summary:

> "In summary, decisions about control of human specimens should turn on the ethical principle of respect for persons, which is embraced by a stewardship, not an ownership model. If we are to realize the promises of this most exciting time in biomedical and epidemiologic research, these decisions must have their foundations within an ethical, not legal framework, motivating all stakeholders in the scientific process."

In summary, patients should not simply assume that they own their stem cells that are in the possession of a for-profit company or a university/non-profit entity. This conclusion unfortunately is very much contrary to what most stem cell patients have told me that they believe.

The possibility that patients may in fact not own their stem cells is increased when companies modify the stem cells (e.g. grow them in culture) to create a new stem cell product that is distinct from the endogenous stem cells. It is also possible that some stem cell clinics require as a condition for receiving an experimental procedure that patients sign a waiver assigning all commercial rights to the stem cells to the company. Because almost no stem cell companies (even those we think of as mostly good citizens in the field) will publicly release the consent forms that they make patients sign,[xv] it is difficult to know what rights patients retain to their own cells or products made from them. The safest assumption is that patients have few rights to their isolated stem cells.

Regardless of ownership, patients' stem cells may also end up being unavailable and out of the reach of patients for other reasons. For example, in Texas a conflict arose between stem cell clinic Celltex and its partner, Human Biostar Inc. (HBI) that impacts patients.

Celltex and HBI had been working together to isolate and grow stem cells in culture. The expanded stem cells of hundreds of patients were then banked in a lab. HBI had been taking care of the laboratory-related aspects of the process including the stem cell cryopreservation and banking. The two companies ended up in conflict, filing suit against each other,[xvi] and HBI moved the entire stem cell bank consisting of more than 200 patient samples to a different location where the cells were for a time inaccessible to Celltex and the patients themselves.

While the cells today are apparently available to patients with certain conditions attached, to my knowledge the long-term status remains not entirely resolved.[xvii] This case serves to illustrate how once a company has possession of your stem cells, unpredictable things can happen that lead you to have control of your own cells taken from you.

[xv]http://stemcellassays.com/2012/12/cells-weekly-december-30-2012/
[xvi]http://www.bizjournals.com/houston/blog/2012/12/celltex-human-biostar-plot-thickens.html
[xvii]http://www.ipscell.com/2012/12/texas-judge-issues-complicated-restraining-order-in-celltex-v-rnl-biohuman-biostar-tussle/

Reason 7: Untrained doctors

In the previous chapter I discussed the unethical practice whereby some inadequately trained physicians are routinely transplanting stem cells into patients. All medical procedures have some risks, but such risks increase dramatically when the doctor performing the action is not trained to conduct it.

When patients need to get a specific procedure done for a given medical reason, they rightly seek out the expert in that area. If you have heart trouble, you go to a cardiologist with the best academic credentials. If you have a stomach problem, you got to a gastroenterologist. When I had prostate cancer in 2009, I looked for the best prostate cancer surgeon.

Yet somehow many patients in the stem cell field often are seemingly okay with greatly lowering their expectations for the training of their doctors. Part of the problem is that there is no official medical specialty in stem cells. Additionally, it is a major concern that stem cell doctors too often start treating patients even though they themselves know they are not adequately trained.

An untrained doctor equals danger. In a recent paper,[xviii] I have called for the creation of academic physician training programs in stem cells (see the curriculum in Figure 8.2). I hope that such programs will be implemented leading to a whole new generation of doctors who truly are specialists in stem cells [4].

Reason 8: The unknown

While stem cell medicine has been around for decades in the form of bone marrow transplants as discussed earlier in this book, there have not been other stem cell treatments that are as common or approved by regulators. In fact, the stem cell field as a whole is a new type of medicine. Stem cell procedures are by and large unknown territory for doctors, regulators, and patients, which means that we just do not know much about them. You might say that there are risks of unknown

---

[xviii]http://www.ncbi.nlm.nih.gov/pubmed/23477401

problems with any medical therapy, but one should keep in mind that generally therapies are rigorously studied for many years before they are used routinely in patients. That is often not the case with stem cells sold by non-compliant clinics so the realm of the unknown is far greater.

A reason some patients consider a high-risk stem cell treatment: The risk of doing nothing

Some of the patients who contact me are in a position where they have decided that getting an experimental, even unlicensed stem cell procedure is the right decision for them. What is their reason? They are facing a terminal or otherwise devastating disease for which they and their physician believe there is no other available option.

They have decided that the potential risks of such a stem cell procedure are outweighed by the risks of doing nothing. I cannot dispute such an argument. But if someone is considering getting a stem cell procedure for this reason, I would recommend that first they do their best to look for an FDA-approved clinical trial at the great clinicaltrials.gov website.[xix] While it is by definition uncertain if the trial itself would be helpful (and it likely has its own risks), at least you will almost certainly be treated ethically by trained physicians, you will not be charged exorbitant fees for participation, and the trial personnel will follow up on you.

This all does not always happen perfectly even in clinical trials, but your odds of being treated overall in an ethical manner are far greater in a compliant clinical trial. In addition through an FDA-approved clinical trial data will be collected and put into the public domain to help future patients.

Summary

I believe that patients receiving stem cell procedures should have inherent rights that I have outlined in this chapter. Part of the need for such rights is that patients are sometimes in a vulnerable position that

---

[xix]http://www.clinicaltrials.gov

makes them subject to unethical behavior by certain providers. Of course many providers are ethical and have the patients' best interests at heart.

Stem cells as innovative, cutting edge technologies also pose unique risks. The relationship between new medical technologies and patient risk can be illustrated by the case of LASIK (Laser-Assisted in Situ Keratomileusis) eye surgery, which enhances patient's vision but also has risks. Would you want to be one of the first patients or even the hundredth patient who ever had their eye zapped for LASIK? I would not because there is a learning curve not just for doctors, but also for whole areas of medicine. Ideally, I would not want to be a patient when an area of medicine is right at the beginning of the learning curve when there are so many unknowns. The same is true of so many stem cell procedures.

A very good question then comes to mind: So who are the first ones to get innovative, experimental therapies?

Many times the first people participating in clinical trials of new therapies and receiving innovative procedures are those who consciously and willingly take a risk. They may be quite sick or even terminally ill. I think they are heroes. My top concern specifically with high-risk procedures offered by for-profit, non-compliant stem cell clinics is that the patients involved are not made aware of just how risky the interventions may be and do not give a true informed consent to be part of an experiment because the providers hide the fact that the procedures are experimental.

I do want to stress that what is known about many stem cell treatments being studied in a compliant manner makes me very excited for their future in medicine. Patients keeping the facts and questions outlined in this chapter in mind have at least a better chance of going into the decision-making process with more information and a realistic sense of what to expect. They should also advocate for their rights including those in the Stem Cell Patient Bill of Rights.

Important Advisory

The chapter above is for information only and is not medical advice. Patients should make medical decisions in consultation with their personal physicians.

References

1. Skloot, R (2010) *The immortal life of Henrietta Lacks.* 1st ed. Crown Publishers.
2. Capps, BJAV Campbell (2010) *Contested cells: global perspectives on the stem cell debate.* Imperial College Press; Distributed by World Scientific Pub.
3. Dressler, LG (2007) Biospecimen "ownership": counterpoint. *Cancer epidemiology, biomarkers & prevention: a publication of the American Association for Cancer Research, cosponsored by the American Society of Preventive Oncology.* **16**:2:190-1.
4. Knoepfler, PS (2013) Call for fellowship programs in stem cell-based regenerative and cellular medicine: new stem cell training is essential for physicians. *Regenerative medicine.* **8**:2:223-5.

Chapter 10

Are We There Yet? How Stem Cells Might Work to Treat Specific Diseases

One of the hardest things about a thrilling new technology still in development is waiting for it to become a reality. This impatience is definitely evoked with emerging stem cell-based regenerative medicine and cellular therapies. With stem cell technology we are far enough along in this revolution to make an educated guess as to how it might work to treat specific diseases. In some cases the already ongoing or planned clinical trials using stem cells for specific diseases also more definitively point the way. Here in this Chapter I discuss potential stem cell applications for some specific diseases (listed in alphabetical order). In some cases these applications are based on the approaches to use stem cells that were discussed in a more general context in Chapter 3.

Alzheimer's Disease (AD)

Alzheimer's Disease (AD) is one of the most devastating illnesses. It destroys the brain, which shrinks over time as the disease progresses.

The toll of AD is not only measured in hundreds of billions of dollars in health care costs and millions of deaths, but also in personal and family tragedy that comes with the severe loss of memory that accompanies it.

Remarkably, scientists and doctors are getting better at predicting who has pre-clinical AD or who will ultimately get AD before patients are even symptomatic. I have to wonder, though, would I want to know I will get AD if doctors have no treatment for it? At this time nobody really knows what causes AD. There are also no known convincing ways to treat or prevent it either. **However, a number of avenues provide hope for the future.**

For example, the *New York Times* published an article about a clinical trial being conducted on a Colombian family that has a strong genetic predisposition to AD.[i] Scientists are testing a treatment on this family using an antibody-based drug called Crenezumab. The drug is an antibody that has as its target the distinctive plaques that form in the AD brain even before the disease becomes clinically apparent. Many other drugs are being developed as well, but an overriding challenge is that, as mentioned above, we do not truly understand AD in the same way that we understand other diseases. For this reason, further research is essential.

Another possible approach to treat AD is through stem cell-based regenerative medicine therapies. There are three key possible approaches to using stem cells to treat AD:

Regrow brain cells via cell therapy. One avenue is to use stem cells to regenerate or regrow diseased parts of the brain. This approach is what people most commonly think of when they conceive of treating AD with stem cells. The problem with this approach is that the architecture of the brain is physically integral to memory so even if we could grow a fresh, young part of the brain to replace one ravaged by AD, there would be no memories there. It would be like wiping the slate clean. In theory perhaps the person could make new memories going forward in life that could be remembered or they could be re-educated, but this is not what most people imagine as a successful treatment for AD.

Heal with immunomodulation. Another approach is to use stem cells such as MSCs not as rebuilding agents, but rather as healers of the existing brain tissue. In this way of thinking, MSC could heal rather than replace neurons for example. MSCs are akin to the natural doctors of the body. They could have anti-inflammatory and other powers that might ameliorate AD.

Drug delivery. A third concept is using stem cells such as MSCs as drug delivery agents. So for example, instead of giving Crenezumab or some other drug systemically, it is possible that stem cells could directly

---

[i]http://www.nytimes.com/2012/05/16/health/research/prevention-is-goal-of-alzheimers-drug-trial.html?ref=health&_r=0

deliver a drug (e.g. one that targets plaques the way that Crenezumab does) within the brain from cell-to-cell far more effectively than a drug given systemically.

Some of these same kinds of approaches might be applicable to other diseases as well. However, all of them might be stymied to some degree by the potentially harsh or even cytotoxic environment of the AD brain, which may kill transplanted cells before they had a chance to do anything positive.

There are eight clinical trials listed in the national database for Alzheimer's and stem cells.[ii]

Amyotrophic Lateral Sclerosis (ALS)

Amyotrophic lateral sclerosis (ALS), also previously known as Lou Gehrig's Disease, is a fatal, motor neuron disease without any known effective treatment or cure. The potential use of stem cells to treat ALS is therefore a very promising possibility.

ALS causes a variety of symptoms of muscle weakness and atrophy including difficulty speaking, swallowing, and breathing. There are thought to be a variety of causes of ALS, which for the most part remain unknown. However, the discovery that some ALS patients have a mutation in a specific gene called superoxide dismutase (SOD) was a potential breakthrough. Importantly, the SOD protein is a cellular detoxification enzyme that tackles free radicals. This suggests that one potential molecular and cellular cause of ALS might be damage to stem cells and other kinds of cells.

However, in most cases the cause of ALS is unclear.

The main way in which stem cell treatments are thought to potentially be helpful in treating ALS is through generating healthy new motor neurons via cell replacement. The company NeuralStem is conducting an ALS clinical trial using transplantation of spinal cord-derived stem cells.[iii]

[ii]http://clinicaltrials.gov/ct2/results?term=alzheimer%27s+AND+stem+cells&Search=Search

[iii]http://clinicaltrials.gov/ct2/show/NCT01348451?term=neuralstem&rank=4

Arthritis

Can stem cells treat the different forms of arthritis that plague hundreds of millions of people across the globe?

A couple years back I did a post in my disease focus series on my blog on the potential of stem cells to be used as treatments for osteoarthritis (OA).[iv] OA affects approximately 30 million people in the US alone and fully one-third of all people over the age of 65. It leads to loss of cartilage in joints such as the knee, where a person can end up with bone on bone.

Almost 1% of all people will get the other main form of arthritis, rheumatoid arthritis, at some point during their lives.

Current treatments for arthritis are suboptimal. For example, there is in fact no current therapy to prevent cartilage deterioration in OA. At this time, therapies for OA are based on systemic immunosuppressive drugs that are less than ideal and have many side effects. The stem cell field continues to advance and I remain convinced that in the future OA as well as rheumatoid arthritis will be successfully treated using stem cell technology.

There is reason for optimism on the stem cell front for arthritis as there are currently 58 clinical trials listed for the search "arthritis" and "stem cells" on the global database.[v]

How might stem cells treat OA and/or rheumatoid arthritis?

There are two main possibilities.

First, there is cell therapy. Stem cells could be used to replace lost or diseased cartilage in the joints. In other words, stem cells would regenerate a healthy (or at least healthier) joint through actual tissue growth. This is the most promising hope for treating OA using stem cells.

Second, there is immunomodulation. Stem cells might be able to be used to tamp down the overactive immune system and inflammation at least in part responsible for joint destruction, particularly for rheumatoid

---

[iv]http://www.ipscell.com/2010/09/disease-focus-series-osteoarthritis-research-moving-forward/

[v]http://clinicaltrials.gov/ct2/results?term=arthritis+AND+stem+cells

arthritis. Stem cells appear to have immune modulating functions that act in an anti-inflammatory manner. MSCs seem especially promising in this area.

I know that for-profit stem cell clinics are already selling stem cell procedures, usually involving MSCs, for arthritis. At this point I say, "buyer beware". Such procedures are expensive and highly experimental. Patients considering them should use caution.

Autism

Autism affects millions of children in the US alone. It is a perplexing spectrum of disorders with "autism" being an umbrella term for this host of related neurological illnesses. The negative impact of autism on our society transcends economics, but has been estimated at 10s of billions of dollars annually.

There is currently no cure or even validated treatment for autism.

Part of the problem is that scientists do not really understand what causes autism and the different forms of the disease likely have distinct causes. Without an understanding of the causes of autism, it is difficult to treat the disease. Add in the fact that autism is really, as mentioned above, a host of related, yet distinct disorders, and treatment becomes even more challenging. Nonetheless, **the idea of using stem cells to treat autism has gained some traction.**

In fact, a first of its kind clinical trial for stem cell-based treatments of autism started right here in Sacramento in 2012 at Sutter Neuroscience Institute run by Dr. Michael Chez. I am not affiliated with them as I work at UC Davis here in Sacramento.

The clinical trial, reported on the front page of Sacramento's daily newspaper, the Sac Bee, involves giving pediatric patients cord blood stem cells as a potential treatment for autism.[vi]

Some of the children in the study will be given placebo, while others will be given an autologous transplant of their own cord blood

---

[vi]http://www.sacbee.com/2012/08/21/4743150/sutter-neuroscience-institute.html

stem cells that were banked when these kids were born. In this context, no immunosuppression should be needed.

The rationale behind the trial is that the stem cells will do something to repair some kind of underlying damage that is responsible for autism.

From the Sac Bee article:

> "Autism is thought to have multiple risk factors, including genetic, environmental and immunological components.
> It is the immunological component that interests Chez most. Much of his research focuses on the relationship between a child's immune system and the central nervous system. Evidence suggests that some children with autism have dysfunctional immune systems that may damage or delay development of the nervous system."

I do not see clear existing evidence of how this clinical trial might work. In the Sac Bee article, Chez proposes an immune mechanism:

> "Cord blood stem cells may offer ways to modulate or repair the immune systems of these patients who have no obvious reason to become autistic"

I remain quite skeptical about the trial at this point. Six other stem cell-based clinical trials are listed in the national database specifically for autism.[vii]

Cancer

One of the challenges of treating "cancer" is of course that there are scores of kinds of cancer and each one is unique in many ways. However, there are some possible avenues to treat a variety of cancers using stem cells (beyond bone marrow transplantation).

[vii]http://clinicaltrials.gov/ct2/results?term=stem+cells+AND+autism

In one possible indirect approach, the knowledge gained from studies of cancer and cancer stem cells is used to develop targeted therapies against cancer stem cells. For example, new drugs may be identified that cause cancer stem cells to undergo apoptosis.

One particularly provocative new cancer stem cell approach is so-called "differentiation therapy". Cancer stem cells have similarities to normal stem cells, but it seems in many cases that the potency of cancer stem cells to differentiate is impaired. In differentiation therapy, cancer stem cells are forced to differentiate, essentially disarming them. It is possible that in order to unlock the differentiation potential of cancer stem cells that they may need to be reprogrammed first to be more akin to pluripotent stem cells.[viii]

Another notion is to use stem cells as a drug delivery device to direct chemo or radiation therapy (via radioactive isotopes carried in the cells rather than external beam radiation) directly through cell-to-cell contact to kill cancer cells. In this approach, it is hypothesized that the side effects of chemo or radiation would be dramatically reduced compared to traditional approaches involving systemic administration.

Chronic Obstructive Pulmonary Disease (COPD)

Chronic obstructive pulmonary disease (COPD) is a relatively common, often debilitating illness, which has a major impact on the people of the world. In the US alone, COPD costs the country almost $50 billion a year not to mention untold suffering. Most of us know someone who has COPD, which is an umbrella term that includes chronic bronchitis and emphysema.

Researchers are still investigating the causes, but two big ones are smoking and pollution. There are a number of treatments for COPD, but no cure. The treatments, which can include supplemental oxygen, are largely palliative. A number of clinics over the years have offered stem cell treatments for COPD, but these treatments are expensive and it is unclear if they work.

[viii]http://www.ncbi.nlm.nih.gov/pubmed/22998387

Some clinical trials are underway for stem cell treatment of COPD (note some of the trials listed below that pop up with different search terms as of 2013 are the same ones):

For emphysema I found 4 stem cell trials,[ix] although unfortunately none are actively recruiting patients. One of the completed studies, based on only four patients, has results that seem inconclusive to this scientist.[x]

For COPD and stem cells, I found 6 stem cell trials, including 2 actively recruiting new patients.[xi]

For Chronic Obstructive Pulmonary Disease and stem cells as search terms, I found 12 trials[xii] including many that are recruiting, which is quite encouraging.

In principle, how would stem cells be used to treat COPD?

There are at least three ideas about how stem cells might benefit these airway diseases.

First, transplants of stem cells could be used for cell therapy. Stem cells may rebuild healthy respiratory tissue that is diseased or has been destroyed in COPD patients. While this approach is exciting, there is not much data to support it.

Second, stem cells could be used for immunomodulation. In this way of thinking, stem cells may reduce inflammation in the airway alveoli (where respiration occurs) preventing further damage and perhaps tipping the balance toward natural repair. Stem cells may do this through so-called "immunomodulation" functions. For more on immunomodulation see Chapter 3.

Third, stem cells may stimulate the formation of new capillaries (the smallest blood vessels) in the lung leading to tissue repair and better function.

There are risks associated with these kinds of treatments including autoimmune reaction (or immune reaction for an allogeneic transplant

[ix]http://clinicaltrials.gov/ct2/results?term=emphysema+AND+stem+cells&Search=Search
[x]http://clinicaltrials.gov/ct2/show/results/NCT01110252?term=emphysema+AND+stem+cells&rank=1
[xi]http://clinicaltrials.gov/ct2/results?term=stem+cells+AND+COPD&Search=Search
[xii]http://clinicaltrials.gov/ct2/results?term=Stem+cells+AND+Chronic+Obstructive+Pulmonary+Disease&Search=Search

such as cord blood), abnormal growth, infection and, emboli. Barring positive or negative action by the FDA for any given clinic, patients must weigh the burden of their COPD versus the potential risks of unvetted stem cell treatments offered by largely non-compliant clinics all relative to the potential benefit of such treatments. In my opinion, these treatments are not worth the risk today, but others disagree. I do have hope for the future in this area.

HIV/AIDS

The great pandemic of modern history, HIV/AIDS, continues. There are now more than 33 million HIV infected individuals. More than 2 million people died from HIV infection in 2008 alone, approximately 1 out of 6 of these deaths were children younger than 15. HIV/AIDS is one of the most serious health issues in the world.

There remains a troubling misconception among the public that with the advent of anti-viral therapy involving protease inhibitors and different types of reverse transcriptase inhibitors, that HIV/AIDS has become much less of a concern. However, anti-viral therapy is not widely available across the globe, up to half of patients with HIV do not respond optimally to this therapy, drug-resistant strains of HIV exist as HIV rapidly evolves, and other serious HIV-associated health risks (e.g. heart disease) are becoming more evident that shorten the life spans of people infected with HIV even with effective anti-viral treatments. Therefore, research into new treatments for HIV/AIDS is essential.

One possible, relatively new avenue for HIV/AIDS treatment involves cutting edge stem cell approaches. Much of this impressive research is going on here in California funded by CIRM. There is a powerful video produced by CIRM and featuring CIRM Director Jeff Sheehy, discussing the need for more research and these critical, new potential areas of regenerative medicine that offer hope.[xiii]

CIRM is funding research by two disease teams (UCLA and City of Hope) into potential therapies whereby patients could receive treatments

---

[xiii]http://www.youtube.com/watch?v=E6qSisZNAX0&feature=player_embedded

of their own hematopoietic stem cells that have been modified in such a way that the HIV virus cannot infect them or their progeny blood cells. Cells that are resistant to HIV infection would have an advantage over others that do not and would gradually come to constitute the vast majority of cells within the person's immune system. While not every HIV virus would necessarily disappear from the body, many patients treated in this way could be for all intents and purposes be cured.

This stem cell-based approach was inspired by the finding that a leukemia patient, Timothy Brown of San Francisco, who also happened to be infected by HIV, appears to have been cured of both leukemia and HIV by a bone marrow transplant.[xiv] The cure is thought to be due to the fact that the marrow donor from whom Brown received the transplant was naturally resistant to HIV. The donor was homozygous for a mutation in the CCR5 gene. The CCR5 protein is a cellular receptor (a protein on the cell membrane surface) that is exploited by HIV, which uses it in a manner akin to a door to get into cells. The naturally occurring CCR5 mutation appears to in effect 'change the locks' on cell membranes so HIV cannot enter cells, rendering the blood cells immune to the virus.

Other possible stem cell-based approaches to attacking the HIV virus include efforts to teach the immune system to hone in on the HIV virus and kill it more effectively. For the vast majority of people, the immune system is not very effective at battling HIV so such an immune-enhancing treatment could be strongly beneficial.

HIV is not going away, the number of people infected continues to grow, and its propensity to evolve rapidly could mean the emergence of more drug resistant strains. According to the World Health Organization (WHO), the number of people dying from AIDS has not significantly decreased around the world in recent years even with the advent of anti-viral therapies.[xv] The bottom line is that it is crucial that we continue to fight this disease and stem cell-based approaches to treating HIV/AIDS bring hope to millions of people.

[xiv] http://www.nytimes.com/2011/11/29/health/new-hope-of-a-cure-for-hiv.html?pagewanted=all&_r=0
[xv] http://www.who.int/hiv/data/global_data/en/index.html

Huntington's Disease

Huntington's Disease (HD) is a genetic disorder characterized by progressive neurological problems caused by neurodegeneration. The cause of HD is spectrum of mutations in a gene that was named "Huntingtin". The exact mechanism by which these mutations cause HD remains somewhat unclear, but the mutated Huntingtin protein is toxic.

The mutated Huntingtin gene and protein are very attractive therapeutic targets and I hope this line of research pays off in a treatment or cure for HD. How might this work? Stem cells seem to be ideal drug delivery devices to lower levels of harmful factors such as the mutated Huntingtin protein, an area strongly supported by CIRM funding.[xvi]

More broadly, researchers have developed molecular medicines that reduce the levels of RNA or protein of specific factors. Stem cells seem to be ideal delivery mechanisms to get the drugs in the right place, as discussed in Chapter 3. Research is underway including right here at our UC Davis Institute for Regenerative Cures to use stem cells to deliver these smart medicines to lower the levels of harmful factors such as the Huntington's protein. In principle the same approach could be used to lower the levels of other harmful molecules in the body such as those associated with Alzheimer's Disease.

Multiple Sclerosis

Multiple sclerosis (MS) is an autoimmune disease in which the immune system attacks its own nervous system. MS is a very serious health problem globally as about 400,000 people have MS in just the US alone and more than 2 million worldwide suffer from the disease. **Almost all of us know someone who has MS.** It is a common disease with a huge negative impact. <u>New treatments are desperately needed and stem cells provide hope.</u>

In patients with MS, the immune system mistakenly attacks the insulation, called myelin, surrounding nerves. It therefore belongs to a

---

[xvi]http://www.cirm.ca.gov/our-funding/awards/msc-engineered-produce-bdnf-treatment-huntingtons-disease-1

class of disorders called demyelinating diseases. This damage disrupts the function of the nerves in profound ways. The symptoms are diverse, but often the disease first manifests as tingling and numbness, weakness in arms or legs, unusual changes in vision, or changes in cognition. More info about the disease can be found at the National MS website.[xvii]

There is no known cure for MS and while some medications are helpful, they can have side effects and certain medications may do more harm than good. In rare cases the disease progresses despite medication. Some MS patients seek out alternative medicine therapies including stem cells interventions.

MS patients regularly contact me and ask me questions about the potential of stem cells to be used for MS.

Do stem cells have promise for MS?

What about clinics offering stem cell treatments now?

There is a great deal of stem cell research ongoing for the treatment of MS that has promise. On the clinical trials website as of 2013 there are 30 studies listed for a search of "stem cells" and "multiple sclerosis", 10 more than just about a year ago in 2012, which is reason for hope.

However, at this time, although a number of clinics in the US and internationally claim that they have effective stem cell treatments for MS (most often using MSCs) and sell them to MS patients, I believe that the science is just not there to support such claims yet. Still I see ads on the Internet claiming to provide effective stem cell treatments for MS, but inevitably they lead to dubious clinics.

More research is needed, particularly FDA approved clinical trials such as those I mentioned above. I would recommend that patients talk to their personal physicians and if medication is not working satisfactorily, perhaps first consider a clinical trial rather than a dubious treatment at a clinic.

Theoretically how might stem cells help MS?

I can see three possible ways.

One way MSCs might help MS is through immunomodulation. This is the predominant approach being sold to MS patients by

---

[xvii]http://www.nationalmssociety.org/

unlicensed for-profit clinics. More generally MSCs are thought to have the power to potentially turn down the level of activity of the immune system in some patients. In that way MSCs may be able to reduce the autoimmunity and inflammation that leads to cell and tissue damage during MS. You can think of it as transplanted MSCs turning down the thermostat of immunity in the nervous system. There are some potential problems with this theory though. MS is a disease of the nervous system and MSCs transplanted IV never make it to the nervous system at all. Based on this reality, in order for MSCs to work in this hypothetical manner for treating MS, they would have to secrete enough factors into the bloodstream to modulate immune system cell activity generally, an enormous task, or they would have to be transplanted directly into the central nervous system. Since most transplanted MSCs appear to be either removed from the blood (into the lung, kidneys, or liver) or killed within hours or days of transplant, there is not much time for the IV transplanted MSCs to modulate the activity of the immune system either. Even those selling MSC transplants for MS admit that multiple MSC treatments are likely necessary, perhaps for the rest of the patients' lives.

A second approach under investigation is to use MSCs as tools for drug delivery to treat MS. In this way, MSCs might home in on areas of damage in MS and release factors that act as medicines to reduce inflammation right in the zone where it is needed most and promote remyelination. They may also "feed" the injured cells growth factors and pro-survival factors. This approach has promise, but it is still in its infancy and needs much investigation. A big challenge is that the MSCs would have to be directly injected into the brain or spinal cord.

Finally, nervous system stem cells, rather than MSCs, could be used for cell therapy via transplantation into the nervous system to help re-myelinate nerves and repair the damage.

Bone marrow transplantation may also be effective to treat or even cure MS, however this procedure is quite risky and it alone can kill some patients making it arguably only appropriate to even consider for the most extreme cases of MS.

Overall I am optimistic about stem cell treatments helping MS, but it is going to take some years and in my view the largely non-compliant or foreign clinics now offering non-FDA approved treatments for MS should be considered only as an extreme, last ditch effort.

Parkinson's Disease (PD)

Parkinson's Disease (PD) is a neurodegenerative disorder that affects more than a million Americans. Symptoms of PD include movement disorders such as tremor as well as muscle rigidity arising from problems with the function of dopaminergic neurons. The disease is progressive, taking an ever more severe toll on patients as they age.

Although it is established that loss of dopaminergic neurons causes the symptoms of PD, the molecular causes of PD are unknown in almost all cases, which unfortunately presents a research challenge for prevention and treatment. However, a great deal of research is ongoing and I am particularly excited about regenerative medicine approaches to treating PD patients. Research funded by the Michael J. Fox Foundation and by CIRM are both making progress. Stem cell approaches are some of the most promising.

For example, reporting their findings in the journal, *Stem Cells*, a team from the Buck Institute tested the idea of treating PD in an animal model using human iPS cells [2]. They first used the iPS cells to make dopamine-producing neurons. These neurons and/or neural progenitors destined to make these neurons were transplanted into rats that had a chemically induced PD-like disorder. Encouragingly, the transplants improved the PD-like symptoms of the rats during the course of the study. While the PD treatment related results in this study are somewhat preliminary and limited in scope, the findings are nonetheless. This study provides evidence that iPS-cell based therapies could one day lead to a cure or effective treatment for PD, and it would likely require no immunosuppression. Work with embryonic stem cells is also promising.

At least for the apparent 12-week course of this study, another significant aspect is that no teratoma or other tumors were reported, giving reason for hope that iPS cell based treatments can indeed be made safe. One potential issue is whether 12 weeks post-transplantation is long enough to test for teratoma or pre-cancerous growths. Even in immunodeficient mouse models, it sometimes takes up to 6 months or more for teratoma from human embryonic stem cells to develop. A more convincing follow up period in rodents would be of at least one year.

I would also note that Michael J. Fox has stressed recently the promise of other, non-stem cell based therapies as well including innovative drug therapies in development for PD.[xviii]

Spinal Cord Injury (SCI)

More than 1 million Americans are living with a spinal cord injury (SCI). There are a variety of causes including car accidents, which are the most common source of the injury. Other notable causes include falls such as that sustained by jockey Michael Martinez,[xix] MS, and also Transverse Myelitis that struck Cody Unser,[xx] sports injuries, cancer, acts of violence (stabbing, gunshots), and war injury leaving many of our veterans with SCIs.

Christopher and Dana Reeve (see the Reeve Foundation here[xxi]) as well as Don C. Reed[xxii] and Roman Reed[xxiii] have been instrumental in bringing attention to the significance of this injury and the importance of research to develop treatments for SCI.

The range of severity of effects from SCI varies with the location and intensity of the trauma (the higher in the spinal column generally the more severe the injury), but the injuries frequently are profoundly devastating. Only rarely do patients who appear to have serious SCI (e.g. paraplegia) experience a complete recovery and usually signs of recovery would begin within days or a few weeks. Thus, sadly most often "miracle" recoveries are found only in a fictional context rather than the real world.

For example there is the case of the character Matthew Crawley (aka Cousin Matthew) on the hit PBS series, *Downton Abbey*. Crawly suffered

---

[xviii]http://abcnews.go.com/blogs/health/2012/05/18/michael-j-fox-looks-past-stem-cells-in-search-for-parkinsons-cure/

[xix]http://www.nydailynews.com/sports/more-sports/paralyzed-jockey-michael-martinez-holds-hope-adult-stem-cell-treatment-spinal-cord-article-1.192144

[xx]http://www.cufsf.org/

[xxi]http://www.christopherreeve.org/site/c.ddJFKRNoFiG/b.4048063/k.C5D5/Christopher_Reeve_Spinal_Cord_Injury_and_Paralysis_Foundation.htm

[xxii]http://stemcellbattles.wordpress.com/

[xxiii]http://romanreedfoundation.com/

complete paraplegia after a war injury during World War I, and showed no sign of recovery months later. However after more months went by somehow he regained complete function.

Unfortunately, such a spontaneous recovery cannot be expected outside of the TV world of *Downton Abbey.*[xxiv] For that reason, it is imperative that new, stem cell-based treatments for SCI be developed. In order for this to happen, research into SCI and potential regenerative medicine treatments must be adequately funded. There is great excitement about BioTime's (based on a stem cell portfolio previously own by the biotech Geron[xxv]) embryonic stem cell-based clinical trial starting to move forward again. More research is needed as well.

The kind of treatment being pioneered by Hans Keirstead and BioTime/Geron involves creating differentiated spinal cord cells such as oligodendrocytes (oligos), from human embryonic stem cells. The principle behind this approach is that the oligos will aid in healing of the spinal cord. Preclinical work has been promising.

A central element of this treatment, as highlighted by the recent case with Martinez, is that the injury has to be of a certain kind to be treatable using BioTime's approach. Animal models suggest that stem cell treatment will not help injuries that are too severe. In addition, the treatment most likely must be given within 1-2 weeks of the injury. The NIH has a very interesting website on the history of spinal cord injury going back thousands of years.[xxvi]

Another potential goal for stem cell-based regenerative medicine therapies for SCI would be to stimulate regeneration. One challenge with this possible approach is to encourage not only engraftment of a transplant but also appropriate, robust axon growth given the architecture and size of the spinal cord.

Finally, a key hope that stem cell research keeps alive is the development of treatments that could work beyond the first week or two after the injury to treat patients potentially years after they have sustained the SCI.

[xxiv]http://apennedpoint.com/downton-abbeys-flirtation-with-medical-facts/

[xxv]http://www.ipscell.com/2012/11/cirm-comment-on-prospect-of-biotime-buying-geron-stem-cell-program/

[xxvi]http://www.ninds.nih.gov/disorders/sci/detail_sci.htm

Summary

From these examples, I hope you can see the great potential of stem cells to be used for many of the most terrible diseases and injuries facing humanity. You might also note the common threads whereby stem cells are being applied in similar ways for different diseases tracing back to the general approaches discussed in Chapter 3. Based on current trends, even more clinical trials using stem cells will begin in the future, giving reason for even more hope.

Of course the diseases discussed above are not all inclusive because an entire book could be written on that topic alone. The diseases not specifically discussed are highly significant too and by no means should their omission be interpreted otherwise.

Also please note that earlier in the book I already discussed some of the approaches currently being used by other biotech companies for certain diseases. For example, I discussed how Athersys is working to use all the four main stem cell approaches to medicine for a variety of human diseases including ulcerative colitis by immunomodulation (Chapter 8).

In addition, I have discussed the company ACT, which is working to treat the leading cause of blindness, macular degeneration, using a cell therapy and replacement approach. In addition I discussed the work of Viacyte for Diabetes using cell therapy in Chapter 3. In theory Diabetes could also be treated using stem cells for immunomodulation.

For all of us facing life-threatening or life-changing diseases, stem cells offer real hope in the future. It is crucial to educate ourselves and avoid letting extreme overexuberance lead to risk taking with dubious therapies, but at the same time we need all the energy and perseverance that we can get to make the most of stem cells to help as many people as possible.

References

1. Hamza, TH, et al. (2010) Common genetic variation in the HLA region is associated with late-onset sporadic Parkinson's disease. *Nat Genet.* **42**:9:781-5.
2. Swistowski, A, et al. (2010) Efficient generation of functional dopaminergic neurons from human induced pluripotent stem cells under defined conditions. *Stem Cells.* **28**:10:1893-904.

Chapter 11

Stem Cell Cosmetics: More Than Skin Deep?

Stem cells are already becoming big business as entrepreneurs try to tap into the excitement over this new technology to turn a profit. In principle I see nothing wrong with making money from stem cells as long as it is done in an ethical manner that does not exploit patients.

In this chapter I will discuss one of the hottest areas for tapping into the stem cell buzz: stem cell cosmetics. In some specific cases (e.g. breast reconstruction after cancer surgery or treatment of burn injury) there is reason to be hopeful about the technology being applied in a responsible manner to produce future medical benefits. I strongly believe that stem cell cosmetic procedures should be pursued only as evidence-based medicine when performed by physicians who are appropriately trained for treatment of patients who are properly consented.

An Emerging Billion Dollar Industry

Stem cell cosmetics is a relatively new industry that is making many claims often based on little science, but at the same time is of interest to legitimate physicians wanting to help patients. Cosmetics based on stem cells as an industry is already generating tens of millions of dollars. It is poised to rapidly become a billion-dollar a year industry, perhaps within a decade or less.

The FDA is taking notice. In 2012 the FDA warned several cosmetics-related businesses including two physicians who conducted stem cell procedures on patients.[i]

---

[i]http://www.fda.gov/ICECI/EnforcementActions/WarningLetters/2012/ucm297245.htm and http://www.fda.gov/ICECI/EnforcementActions/WarningLetters/2012/ucm301620.htm

How are stem cells used for cosmetic purposes today and how might they be used in the future? I discuss a few examples in depth below.

Stem cell creams

One of the most popular types of stem cell-related cosmetic products today, but ironically the one with the least scientific basis to think it will actually work, is the stem cell cream (aka crème, which sounds fancier and is more expensive). Stem cell creams are claimed to reverse aging. The creams of this kind are intentionally marketed to consumers as somehow having the power of stem cells because in some people's minds the phrase "stem cells" is strongly associated with cutting edge technology and youthfulness. However, there is currently no clear evidence that such stem cell creams actually make skin more youthful, and in part this is why the FDA has taken action.

Most recently the FDA sent a warning letter to Lancome/L'Oreal regarding its anti-aging stem cell creams alleging that the company made unsubstantiated health-related claims.[ii] Interestingly, these particular creams do not have human, mammalian or even animal stem cells in them. They do not have chemicals or products derived from such stem cells as ingredients either.

Instead these stem cell creams apparently have plant stem cell extracts in them. For example, apple stem cell extracts is a common ingredient. How exactly a plant stem cell extract would help human skin become younger remains unclear. There is some vague notion that extracts of stem cells, even plant stem cells, might have some magic elixir-like quality. I suppose one more realistic possibility is that plant stem cell extracts present in the creams could contain growth factors that stimulate endogenous animal skin stem cells, but this seems highly unlikely. Also now emerging on stem cell creams that have secretions of human stem cells in them as well, possibly including growth factors, raising additional safety concerns.

[ii] http://www.fda.gov/ICECI/EnforcementActions/WarningLetters/2012/ucm318809.htm

These creams, many of which are currently for sale at popular retailers, are very expensive. For example, sixteen ounces of one particular stem cell anti-aging product costs approximately $10,000. My recent search for stem cell products available for sale at a common retailer on their website produced about 3-dozen results, all very expensive. When I searched Amazon.com for "stem cell cream" I found more than eight hundred results, and a "stem cell supplements" search produced more than one hundred results of products for sale. This is clearly big business, but sadly supported by little or no science.

Medical stem cell cosmetic procedures

While stem cell creams may be a waste of money as their efficacy is questionable at best, more worrisome from a health and safety perspective are invasive stem cell cosmetic procedures.

Today such procedures include facelifts, breast augmentation, skin rejuvenation, and baldness remedies. The demand for such cosmetic stem cell medical procedures is already exploding so supply will keep up with demand, especially in so lucrative an arena. The range of cosmetic procedures involving stem cells will continue to grow rapidly. I am concerned about some of these stem cell cosmetic procedures and I was one of the first to ring the alarm bell on aspects of this new area.[iii]

In many cases the physicians performing cosmetic procedures with stem cells including transplantation lack any formal training in the use of stem cells or even in stem cell biology. In fact, it is no exaggeration to say that you know more than some of these doctors about stem cell biology and stem cell procedures just from reading this book. And yet they are injecting patients with stem cells. They have ethical and legal responsibilities to protect their patients and follow up with their patients over time to look for side effects. How can they do that properly if they know next to nothing about stem cells?

The ignorance and lack of training of some physicians also makes it impossible for them to conduct a proper and legally required informed

---

[iii]http://www.ipscell.com/2012/02/from-boobs-to-baldness-stem-cells-go-cosmetic/

consent with their patients about benefits and risks of stem cell cosmetic procedures. A lack of physician training puts patients at risk, especially combined with the sky-high prices for these procedures incentivizing more and more usually untrained doctors to perform them.

To be clear, some doctors in this area do know their stuff and genuinely want to use stem cell cosmetics to help patients. They take these procedures and training for them quite seriously. I have talked extensively with some of them. I am impressed by their depth of knowledge and very serious approach to this evolving form of cosmetic medicine.

I would also note more generally that there are medical reasons for getting some forms of cosmetic surgery. Further, while cosmetic procedures are not my cup of tea, I can respect the fact that even in the absence of a pressing medical need, some patients make informed choices to get cosmetic procedures that improve their self-esteem and perhaps overall well-being. When appropriately trained physicians perform these procedures on properly consented patients and carefully follow up on their patients, I see no reason to question it. I am a stem cell scientist, not a sociologist.

Hypothetically, new cosmetic procedures using stem cells, particularly if they are conducted in the context of a clinical trial, could help people in some novel ways and seem promising for certain conditions, but there are some concerns even from doctors themselves.

Recommendations from the leading plastic surgery associations on stem cell procedures

Cosmetic surgeons apparently have some reservations overall too on stem cell procedures. A joint position statement in 2011 by the two leading plastic surgery associations, the American Society for Aesthetic Plastic Surgery (ASAPS) and the American Society of Plastic Surgeons (ASPS) was cautious.[iv] Dr. J. Peter Rubin, MD, who chaired the task

---

[iv]http://www.surgery.org/media/news-releases/asaps-and-asps-issue-joint-position-statement-on-stem-cells-and-fat-grafting

force established by ASAPS and ASPS, issued a statement mixing a sense of promise and caution:

> "There are encouraging data from laboratory and clinical studies to suggest that the use of adult stem cells is a very promising field," said Dr. Rubin, "but as our comprehensive review of the current scientific literature shows, the data available today do not substantiate the marketing claims being made to patients seeking aesthetic surgery and aesthetic medical treatments."

The task force made six key recommendations about stem cell cosmetic procedures:

- Terms such as "stem cell therapy" or "stem cell procedure" should only be used in very limited, specific cases.
- The marketing and promotion of stem cell procedures in aesthetic surgery is not adequately supported by clinical evidence at this time.
- Stem cell cosmetic procedures should be conducted within IRB-approved clinical trials.
- The collection and reporting of data on outcomes and safety by any physician performing stem cell therapies is strongly encouraged.
- Stem cell based procedures should be performed in compliance with FDA regulatory guidelines.
- Patients are advised to seek consultation for aesthetic procedures by a surgeon certified by the American Board of Plastic Surgery.[v]

These recommendations are sensible and go a long way to protecting patients. Keep them in mind as I discuss how stem cells are being marketed and used for cosmetic procedures.

---

[v]You can check if a prospective doctor is Board Certified in this area here: http://www.abplsurg.org/moddefault.aspx

Is fat the king of stem cell cosmetics?

When it comes to our diets, a recent mantra is "fat has gotten a bad rap." However, in the stem cell field it is quite different. Fat is king and has been for quite a long time. When I go to conferences, talk to patients, and interact with physicians, I hear so much positive buzz about fat.

The reason that fat is so popular with aspects of the stem cell crowd is that it turns out that fat is a good source of stem cells, MSCs more specifically. MSCs derived from adipose (fat) tissue are called adMSCs. Fat is also relatively easy to take out of the body via liposuction and even that has been scaled down to be now commonly performed as "micro-liposuction" or "micro-lipo" for short.

Sometimes cosmetic doctors use fat as a "filler" to smooth out wrinkles via a process called "fat transfer" whereby fat is moved from one part of the body where it is not wanted (e.g. abdomen) to a place where it is hoped to do some good (the face).

Doctors can learn how to do micro-lipo and buy the equipment for their office; together this equips them to in theory take fat from almost any patient. If the doctor then buys a readily available kit or device to isolate adMSCs from fat, this doctor can in theory start performing lucrative stem cell procedures fairly quickly. But without extensive training, education, and knowledge, such doctors are putting their patients at risk and indeed their own clinical practices at great jeopardy from litigation should they make mistakes.

How are Stem Cells Isolated from Fat?

In many physicians' offices where adMSCs are used clinically, a lab sited in the clinic manually isolates the stem cells from the fat. Apparently other clinics offering adMSC-related cosmetic procedures use two devices, Celution and StemSource, made by Cytori Therapeutics Inc. to process the patient samples to isolate adMSCs for clinical use.

The FDA ruled that the Cytori devices require more thorough evaluation including human clinical trials prior to release to the market.

While Cytori appealed the ruling, the US Court of Appeals upheld the FDA's position in March of 2013.[vi]

The devices sell for $100,000 each and are used by a number of plastic surgeons. An *Associated Press* article provided some valuable background on the company's position (as communicated by CFO, Mark Saad) on the off-label use of their devices for potentially non-compliant stem cell procedures:

> "Cytori stresses that it does not market its products in the U.S. for use in stem cell procedures. However, the company has previously sold its $100,000 devices to plastic surgeons across the U.S. for use as 'laboratory equipment' for research, a gray area that is not overseen by the FDA.

> Surgeons in Los Angeles, Miami and elsewhere claim to have used Cytori-processed cells to perform 'stem cell facelifts,' which they market as an alternative to the incisions and implants of traditional plastic surgery. But there are few studies to support such claims, and the FDA has not approved any therapies using stem cells for cosmetic use.

> Saad said Cytori is not responsible for how researchers use the device and that the company is cooperating as much as possible with the FDA.

> "Do we have 100 percent control over what third party doctors do with things they find? Of course not," Saad said. "People have the ability, under the practice of medicine, to do a variety of things and it's up to their medical boards to review them."

[vi]http://www.bloomberg.com/news/2013-03-22/cytori-loses-bid-to-overturn-fda-bar-on-stem-cell-devices.html

I would argue that it is in the best interests of a device manufacturer that is aware of the unapproved use of its devices in non-compliant stem cell procedures to take some steps to protect patients and try to reduce such non-compliant use, even if it is not technically legally required to do so.

Two fat acronyms: SVF and CAL

Two of the hottest acronyms in the for-profit stem cell world remain unknown to most academic stem cell scientists: SVF and CAL.

What do these acronyms stand for and what is the story behind each one?

SVF is an acronym that stands for "stromal vascular fraction". Another group has called a very similar product by the name adipose tissue-derived stem and regenerative cells (ADRCs), but SVF is the name that has caught on so I will use it here [1]. SVF is a laboratory derivation of elements of fat tissue via a process described below.

A physician typically does liposuction or micro-lipo to aspirate fat out of a patient's body, most likely their abdomen. They collect a volume about equal to a 16-ounce bottle of soda (500ml).

The clinic then treats the fat tissue with an enzyme called collagenase that breaks apart tissues to dissociate the fat. They then centrifuge the fat into fractions based on density. The top, least dense fraction is fat, which is thrown away. Then there is a fraction made up of fluid and perhaps some blood plasma. This is also discarded as biohazardous waste.

Finally, at the bottom of the tube is a pellet of cells and other elements, which are denser than fat or liquid. This bottom pellet is called the "Stromal Vascular Fraction" or SVF. Figure 11.1 outlines the process of making SVF. A helpful review paper also details specific aspects of the process for making SVF as follows [2]:

> "In humans and mice, the stromal vascular fraction
> (SVF) is a heterogeneous mixture of cells isolated
> by enzymatic dissociation of adipose tissue followed
> by gradient centrifugation in order to remove the

differentiated adipocytes, which float over the aqueous layer. The pellet of SVF cells contains multipotent mesenchymal cells, which are typically referred to as adipose derived stem/stromal/progenitor cells (ASC)."

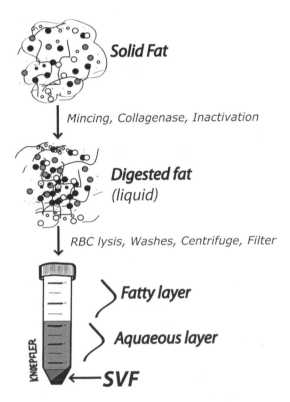

Figure 11.1. Brief overview of the process used to make the SVF stem cell product. Note that the process and the SVF end products vary widely in composition in different clinics and labs. Briefly, fat (adipose) tissue isolated by liposuction is cooled, minced, and treated with an enzyme called collagenase that liquefies the fat and breaks apart connective tissue. The enzyme is then usually inactivated using the patient's own serum that contains enzyme inhibitors (otherwise the enzyme could eventually kill the cells). The Red Blood Cells (RBCs) in the fat are lysed, the preparation is washed with saline, and then spun in a centrifuge separating out into 3 main layers. The SVF is the densest so it is at the bottom of the tube. The SVF is isolated, filtered, and diluted into saline before transplantation or propagation in a lab.

The SVF is not a naturally occurring cellular compilation, but rather a laboratory-constructed conglomeration of a host of cell types including MSCs, pre-adipocytes (fat precursor cells), endothelial and pre-endothelial cells, and stromal cells. There are almost certainly other, unidentified cells types present as well. Also in the SVF mix are non-cellular elements that simply by their density being similar to cells get co-purified with the cells. Such non-cellular elements may not be removed by subsequent washes and could secrete growth factors.

Under current guidelines, SVF is a drug subject to regulation by the FDA. However, many physicians disagree with this classification and there continues to be a lively debate over whether SVF should be regulated as a drug or a tissue. It is possible that the FDA may revise its guidelines to ultimately classify SVF not as a drug in the future, but today it is definitely considered a drug by the FDA. For example, an inquiry by a cosmetic practice to the FDA[vii] over whether manipulated fat such as SVF is a drug yielded a response that indeed the product is a 351 drug (recall our discussion of the difference between 351 and 361 products in Chapter 7).

SVF can be cultured in a lab to expand the cell numbers prior to transplantation into patients or be directly injected once diluted in saline. Culturing seems to inherently change the properties of the SVF cellular population as evidenced by altered expression of surface marker proteins (decreased CD34 and increased CD105; these are membrane proteins of the type that we discussed in Chapter 5 that go by names starting with the CD acronym that stands for "cluster of differentiation"). Such culturing would also appear to inherently alter the product in many other ways that are not clearly understood.

The acronym CAL stands for Cell-Assisted Lipotransfer. It is a procedure whereby fat tissue mixed with stem cells is transplanted into patients as an autologous therapy. Dr. Kotaro Yoshimura pioneered CAL [3]. Fat that is isolated by micro-lipo is used to produce SVF, which is

---

[vii]http://www.cosmeticsurg.net/blog/2012/01/11/fda-stem-cells-from-your-own-fat-are-a-drug/ . Note that the actual FDA correspondence letter is helpfully included at the bottom of that website for reference.

then mixed with remaining fat from the micro-lip to generate a fat product that is enriched for stem cells and other components of SVF.

The basic rationale behind CAL would seem to be that it is a stem cell boosted-fat transfer. CAL is also a biological drug that should be regulated by the FDA, but often physicians doing CAL have no Investigational New Drug (IND) or other approval from the FDA.

Even so, both SVF and CAL are now commonly used around the world and in the US, largely without regulatory oversight. These procedures and products need further study in clinical trials as well as evaluation by regulators.

Fat chance? Hurdles to clinical use of fat stem cells

As much as there is great excitement about SVF and CAL in certain crowds, there are important potential challenges to their use beyond the debate over their regulation by the FDA as drugs in the US. Below, I outline the key biological hurdles.

SVF and CAL heterogeneity. As discussed further later in this chapter, not all fat is created equal, but in addition it would seem that every preparation of SVF and every CAL procedure will be different because of experimental variables between different labs and physicians. Therefore when a customer goes in to get a procedure based on SVF or CAL, in each case the procedure could be quite different beyond the inherent differences intrinsic to each patient.

Impurity. Another issue with fat-related stem cell procedures is that the preparations of various stem cell-related products from fat are often impure, containing a host of different cells and other factors [4]. The risks from impurities seem quite real and significant. For example, in one case a patient received an autologous stem cell transplant leading to hematuria (blood in the urine) and had large masses in the kidney thought to be due to the unintended actions of hematopoietic stem cells present in the preparation [5].

Fibrosis. Another serious risk from fat-based cosmetic procedures is that the stem cell/fat tissue transplantation may lead to fibrosis, a form of undesired growth due to expansion of fibroblasts. Under certain conditions of CAL in the breast, fibrosis has been observed to follow transplantation of adMSCs leading to formation of hard, scar-like tissue, a negative clinical outcome [6]. Fibrosis is also possible with other forms of MSC-based transplants as MSCs will readily differentiate into fibroblasts. Fibrosis caused by an MSC, SVF, or CAL transplant could have more than cosmetically unsatisfactory outcomes. For example, two cases of liver fibrosis caused by such transplants raise the concern of significant negative health impacts on patients [7, 8].

Transplanted cell death. It is now fairly widely accepted that a substantial percentage of transplanted stem cells, including in adipose-related procedures such as those involving MSCs, relatively rapidly dies after introduction into the patient [9]. When MSCs and fat tissue as well as other types of stem cells die inside a recipient patient there is the potential for harm to that patient. Dead and dying stem cells and tissues release unique growth factors, some of which can cause fibrosis (see above) and inflammation that is harmful. It is also possible that larger scale immune reactions could occur.

Fat friends: stimulation of endogenous cancer cells? Fat stem cells are secretion machines. After transplantation, they produce a host of factors that can powerfully impact the behavior of the endogenous cells around them. Often times this factor secretion is imagined in a positive light to heal, but potentially fat stem cells such as MSCs can do harm in this way too.

Two recent research papers point to the ability of fat stem cells to strongly stimulate cancer cell growth in co-culture experiments [10, 11]. What this mean is that when MSCs and cancer cells are grown together, the cancer cells grow dramatically faster than they do without the MSCs along for the ride in the culture dish. Therefore, if a patient who received an AdMSC transplant had existing pre-cancerous cells in the vicinity, it is possible that the transplant might stimulate their growth and increase patient risk in this way.

Not all fat is created equal. All over the US and the world doctors are doing fat transfer procedures on patients by moving fat or adMSCs from one place in the body to another. Some of these physicians see fat and adMSCs, no matter their source, as some kind of universal building material for the body. Squirt it here. Squirt it there. Squirt it everywhere! Good stuff.

However, it is not that simple. Recent studies suggest that not all fat is created equal[viii] so that taking abdominal fat and putting it, for example, into the face or other locations could pose unknown risks. We just do not know how some fat from one place will behave in its new home in the long run. The most likely negative outcome is that the fat or stem cells from fat will be unhappy and die in its new home because of the trauma of the transplant or the lack of a proper niche, but many questions remain even as the number of these procedures being conducted continues to skyrocket.

Stem cell facelifts

Stem cell facelifts using injections of adMSCs or of SVF into the face or CAL procedures into the face of patients to try to look younger are growing in popularity. In many cases the goal is to reverse age-related facial atrophy [12], while in some situations the objective is to address other related aging issues. In addition, stem cell procedures on the face may have more pressing medical needs to address in the future such as facial injuries from trauma such as that suffered on the battlefield.

Dr. Rubin of the plastic surgery association task force mentioned earlier in this chapter, was quoted in an April 2013 *New York Times* piece[ix] on stem cell facelifts (notably in their fashion and style section, not in the science or health section) about the promise of this technology. One particular striking section of that piece was the following:

> "For now, the task force is urging caution on all aesthetic stem-cell procedures, and a hearty dose of "let the buyer beware." The report states "the marketing and promotion of stem cell procedures in aesthetic surgery is not adequately supported clinical by evidence at this time."

[viii]http://www.medicalnewstoday.com/releases/254885.php
[ix]http://www.nytimes.com/2013/04/04/fashion/the-debate-over-stem-cell-face-lifts.html?pagewanted=all&_r=0

But that is not to say that there isn't potential here. "Stem cells in fat are very powerful releasers of growth factors that enhance tissue healing and can induce the growth of new blood vessels in the tissue," Dr. Rubin said. His lab is in the midst of a clinical trial, financed by the National Institutes of Health, on the use of stem-cell-enhanced fat grafting versus nonenhanced fat grafting for treating facial deformities on wounded soldiers. When the trial is complete, the results will help either bolster or diminish the case for procedures like the stem-cell face-lift."

I think the mantra "let the buyer beware" is indeed appropriate in this arena. These procedures, performed both by trained, but also relatively untrained physicians, pose a number of safety concerns related to the obstacles discussed in the last section as well as additional issues. For example, the injected stem cells may not differentiate into the cells/tissues that the physician and patient hope for going into the procedure. MSCs can differentiate into not just fat, but also potentially bone, cartilage, blood vessels, and other cell types.

The patient who got bone in her eye from a stem cell facelift mentioned earlier in this book is perhaps the poster child for caution over such procedures.[x]

A second safety risk is that the cells may leave the site of injection and move around. Recall the discussion in earlier chapters of how stem cells can sometimes be quite migratory. What this means is that stem cells, for example, injected into the skin near the eye, may end up elsewhere in the face or neck. Certainly at least some stem cells also ends up in the blood stream after which they can go anywhere in the body. This is a broader concern than just with facelifts. There are surprisingly little data on the movement of injected stem cells around the body to so-called "off-target" sites.

---

[x]http://www.scientificamerican.com/article.cfm?id=stem-cell-cosmetics

A spoonful of stem cells makes the face go up?

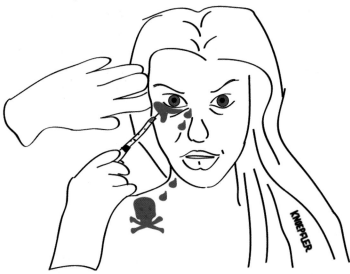

Figure 11.2. More patients are getting cosmetic injections of stem cells or other stem cell-related products such as CAL and SVF into their faces for "stem cell facelifts" or into other body parts such as the breast. These procedures have the potential to cause dangerous effects such as unwanted tissue growth or fibrosis, especially when performed by non-compliant clinics and untrained doctors. Other clinics or cosmetic practices, by contrast, are quite serious about compliance and training, taking a more cautious approach that I view as appropriate.

Another concern is that the cells could grow out of control either to form a benign tumor or a cancer after a cosmetic procedure. While studies would suggest that the risk of such growth with MSCs is quite low, it should not be entirely dismissed as so many clinics do. Fibrosis is also a concern again here in the face as well.

All of the eight reasons to avoid unlicensed stem cell procedures discussed in Chapter 9 also apply here. A broad and serious risk is that there is so little standardizing of how dermatologists and plastic surgeons as well as other doctors are doing these procedures. Combine that with sparse data on the outcomes and we just do not know how any given patient will fare.

In my cartoon in Figure 11.2, I try to capture the risks and emotions of stem cell facelifts visually. One development that could be very helpful is the creation of academic fellowship training programs in cellular and regenerative medicine, something I am actively promoting at this time [13].

Stem cell breast reconstruction and augmentation

There are more potentially medically valuable cosmetic procedures for which stem cells have real promise. Patients recovering from cancer, burn injury and other conditions often greatly benefit from cosmetic procedures. One type of stem cell-based procedure that addresses a medical need is for breast reconstruction after cancer, such as what actress Suzanne Somers self-reported that she recently had performed.

Somers, the actress who played the iconic blonde, Christmas "Chrissy" Snow, in the 70s sitcom *"Three's Company"*, was known back then almost 40 years ago for being a young, sexy actress. Perhaps it is then no surprise that she is now also known for her series of books on staying sexy as one ages and her own line of health products that are sold on her website. She has millions of fans today just as she did decades ago in her twenties. Somers is very interested in stem cells.

A dozen years ago, cancer entered her life as she was diagnosed with breast cancer. Her cancer treatment had side effects that understandably concerned her:

> "Like millions of other women who have been diagnosed with breast cancer, I had to face the numerous daunting decisions about my treatment and recovery. In 2000, I had a lumpectomy and full course of radiation that left me with a withered, nearly pancake breast on the right side (barely a B cup) and my full natural breast on the left side (a D cup)"[xi]

One possible non-stem cell-related option that many women choose in that kind of situation is breast reconstruction that can involve an implant. However, implants (whether filled with saline or silicon) pose

---

[xi]http://www.suzannesomers.com/

definite risks. Fat transfer from one part of the body to the breast to aid in reconstruction is another, relatively newer option.

Somers appears to have had a CAL-like procedure using SVF combined with her fat for an autologous transplant to the breast for reconstruction. The idea is to use a mixture of a woman's own fat and stem cells to reconstruct and literally grow new, healthy breast tissue. As a result, instead of a synthetic implant, the patient in essence has a "real, new" breast composed of her own cells and tissues.

This technology is so new that it is unclear in a general sense how safe and effective it is, but in principle it could work. As with any procedure there are risks.

What could the risks be?

One paper explored the possibility that fat grafting to the breast could increase cancer risk, but concluded that there was no clear evidence of this to date [14]. As mentioned above, leading plastic surgery associations have some concerns about these kinds of procedures and fibrosis is a serious potential side effect.

Somers has a series of videos on another website showing her going through the surgical procedure and during her recovery.[xii] I believe it was very gutsy of her to have the procedure taped.[xiii]

A more general possible concern about this kind of stem cell procedure that has been mentioned to me by people in the stem cell field is that it is increasingly being conducted for patients who do not have compelling disease or injury-related medical needs for it. For example, beyond treatment of cancer patients, the same kind of procedure is apparently being performed more often now for breast augmentation in women who have not had cancer. Other stem cell-related procedures related to stimulating breast growth are being studied as well including an electronic stem cell bra proposed, but unproven to enlarge breasts.[xiv]

If indeed CAL breast augmentation is proven in clinical studies to work and to be at least as safe or safer than implants, then it seems like a

---

[xii]http://www.sexyforever.com/publicsite/suzannes-surgery-video-entry.aspx

[xiii]Note that some of these videos are very graphic medically such as showing surgery and may not be appropriate for all viewers.

[xiv]http://www.stemcellbra.com/

reasonable procedure. But the physicians involved must be properly trained and go through a thorough informed consent process with their patients prior to the treatment.

At this time it remains unknown if the stem cells added to the adipose tissue transplant to the breast make a clinically meaningful difference. Today I would classify these procedures as experimental and the stem cell products that are used are likely to be viewed by the FDA as drugs.

Three clinical trials are listed based on a search for "stem cells" AND "breast reconstruction",[xv] but it seems that Somers' trial at least so far is not currently in that database.

I hope Somers is doing well and wish her the best of health.

Stem cell procedures for baldness

There is reason for some optimism that stem cells might actually treat or cure baldness in the future. Baldness procedures can be about vanity, but not always. Many medical procedures such as radiation treatment for brain cancer or chemo as well as medical conditions such as burns or alopecia cause baldness, strongly affecting the self-esteem and quality of life of millions of patients. In addition, many people simply progressively get balder as they age, not as the result of a disease.

There is reason for hope that stem cells from the skin that make hair might be widely used in the next 10-20 years for treating or even curing baldness. The research to date on this possible application of stem cell technology seems very promising.

How would stem cell procedures for baldness work?

Two main approaches are imagined. First, there is the possibility of autologous stem cell therapy for baldness. Second, there is a very real possibility of a drug stimulating the hair follicle stem cells to be more active, producing more hair. In the former case, research on specialized skin stem cells that can grow hair has been advancing at a rapid clip.[xvi]

[xv] http://www.clinicaltrials.gov/ct2/results?term=stem+cells+AND+breast+reconstruction &Search=Search

[xvi] http://www.nytimes.com/2012/07/29/business/baldness-battle-fought-in-the-follicle.html?_r=0

Today male pattern baldness on the head is often treated with so-called "hair plugs". Doctors move hair from a relatively dense area such as the back of the head into bald regions. Most often the hair survives and grows in its new home, an endogenous stem cell dependent process. In the directly stem cell-based approach for baldness, instead of moving hairs, doctors would transplant hair stem cells into bald regions and the stem cells would grow new hairs from scratch.

Alternatively, doctors may use some of the patient's own stem cells to grow skin with hairs for them in a lab and then transplant those together as a tissue into balding areas of the scalp. If these technologies can be realized, stem cell-based baldness procedures may turn into a multi-billion dollar industry.

Summary

Beyond baldness and breast reconstruction, stem cells are also currently already being offered for many other cosmetic uses under less than ideal scientific contexts.

The area of stem cell cosmetics is booming and is largely unregulated so far. **Until proven safe and effective, cosmetic products or procedures claiming to use stem cells should be viewed as experimental.**

References

1. Feng, Z, et al. (2010) Fresh and cryopreserved, uncultured adipose tissue-derived stem and regenerative cells ameliorate ischemia-reperfusion-induced acute kidney injury. *Nephrology, dialysis, transplantation: official publication of the European Dialysis and Transplant Association - European Renal Association.* **25**:12:3874-84.
2. Scherberich, A, ND Di MaggioKM McNagny (2013) A familiar stranger: CD34 expression and putative functions in SVF cells of adipose tissue. *World journal of stem cells.* **5**:1:1-8.
3. Yoshimura, K, et al. (2008) Cell-assisted lipotransfer for cosmetic breast augmentation: supportive use of adipose-derived stem/stromal cells. *Aesthetic plastic surgery.* **32**:1:48-55; discussion 56-7.
4. Reinders, METJ Rabelink (2010) Adipose tissue-derived stem cells: can impure cell preparations give pure results? *Nephrology, dialysis, transplantation: official*

publication of the European Dialysis and Transplant Association - European Renal Association. **25**:12:3805-7.

5. Thirabanjasak, D, K TantiwongsePS Thorner (2010) Angiomyeloproliferative lesions following autologous stem cell therapy. *Journal of the American Society of Nephrology: JASN.* **21**:7:1218-22.

6. Yoshimura, K, et al. (2008) Ectopic fibrogenesis induced by transplantation of adipose-derived progenitor cell suspension immediately after lipoinjection. *Transplantation.* **85**:12:1868-9.

7. Russo, FP, et al. (2006) The bone marrow functionally contributes to liver fibrosis. *Gastroenterology.* **130**:6:1807-21.

8. di Bonzo, LV, et al. (2008) Human mesenchymal stem cells as a two-edged sword in hepatic regenerative medicine: engraftment and hepatocyte differentiation versus profibrogenic potential. *Gut.* **57**:2:223-31.

9. Eto, H, et al. (2012) The fate of adipocytes after nonvascularized fat grafting: evidence of early death and replacement of adipocytes. *Plastic and reconstructive surgery.* **129**:5:1081-92.

10. Yu, JM, et al. (2008) Mesenchymal stem cells derived from human adipose tissues favor tumor cell growth in vivo. *Stem cells and development.* **17**:3:463-73.

11. Martin-Padura, I, et al. (2012) The white adipose tissue used in lipotransfer procedures is a rich reservoir of CD34+ progenitors able to promote cancer progression. *Cancer research.* **72**:1:325-34.

12. Yoshimura, K, et al. (2008) Cell-assisted lipotransfer for facial lipoatrophy: efficacy of clinical use of adipose-derived stem cells. *Dermatologic surgery: official publication for American Society for Dermatologic Surgery [et al.].* **34**:9:1178-85.

13. Knoepfler, PS (2013) Call for fellowship programs in stem cell-based regenerative and cellular medicine: new stem cell training is essential for physicians. *Regenerative medicine.* **8**:2:223-5.

14. Fraser, JK, MH HedrickSR Cohen (2011) Oncologic risks of autologous fat grafting to the breast. *Aesthetic surgery journal / the American Society for Aesthetic Plastic surgery.* **31**:1:68-75.

Chapter 12

Stem Cell Tests for Humanity

Many ethical issues surround stem cell research and technology. How society handles these controversial stem cell areas has great importance not only for science, but also the future of humanity.

As discussed in Chapter 8 and throughout this book, there are ethical issues on stem cell commercialization, but there are also broader ethical issues related to stem cells that are not so directly related just to commercialization. It is the latter that are the focus of this chapter.

For a decade the main ethical debate in the stem cell field has been over human embryonic stem cells and that is discussed in this chapter. However, there are a number of other important ethical questions related to stem cells including some that are coming to the forefront today.

For example, some developing areas in the stem cell field literally may change what it means to be a human being via stem cell-related assisted reproduction technologies. The public may not realize how stem cell technology has brought the kind of manipulated laboratory-based human reproduction in *Brave New World* much closer to reality.

Embryonic Stem Cells: When Does a Human Life Begin and Who Decides?

At the heart of the embryonic stem cell debate is the question of when human life begins.

I do not claim to know for sure when the life of a human being starts, but I do have some thoughts on the topic. In addition, I believe I know for myself when life does *not* begin: at conception and at birth. For me it is somewhere in between. Most scientists are afraid to talk publicly about this question and probably for good reason because of its controversial nature.

There is no one "right" answer as to when human life begins. For many people in our world, they desire some authority to tell them the answer. Who decides when a human being begins? It would seem there are a handful of key possible authorities that people turn to, rightly or wrongly, on the question of when human life begins.

Religious authorities

Importantly, while in Christianity, many ministers today argue that human life begins at conception, leaders in other religions have different views generally pointing towards a later start for a human being. There is no one "right" religious answer to the question of when life begins.

Ethical authorities

Some people turn to ethicists on this question of life. I have interacted over the years with a few people who are not particularly religious, but who nonetheless believe that human life begins at conception and that embryonic stem cell research is unethical because it is killing a human being. Many other ethicists, however, believe life begins later. A number of patient advocates highlight the importance of embryonic stem cell research as ethical because it may save millions of lives and reduce human suffering using blastocysts that would otherwise be thrown away.

Doctors

A number of people think that because of their medical training that doctors have a unique authority to somehow know when life begins for human beings. However, in my own informal survey of doctors, there was no consensus.

Scientists

Other people turn to scientists hoping for some kind of scientific proof of when life begins. As a scientist myself, I would argue that we do not have the answer because there is no scientific answer to this question. Further, clearly there is no experiment to determine when life begins although one scientist argued there was and I rebutted her claims.[i] There is no equation like $E=MC^2$ for defining the moment when a human life begins as opposed to a living human cell.

Legal authorities

While others turn to judges and legal scholars for the answer to the question of when life begins, I am not convinced they have any better answers than anyone else. To my knowledge in the US there is no federal law on when life begins either, however there are state laws on fetal homicide that define an unborn fetus as a person. A wider law on when life begins (e.g. Proposed personhood laws in the US that define life at conception, but which have generally failed to be approved) could negatively influence pregnant women in many ways as well as people more broadly related to contraception, for example. In fact, there is no "the answer", whether scientific or not, which applies to everyone.

When Do Cells Become People and a Human Being's Life Begins?

There are seven main possibilities when the life of a human being might start: (1), before conception (yes, you read that right), (2) at conception, (3) at implantation, (4) when the heart starts beating, (5) when distinctively human, organized brain activity begins, (6) when the fetus can survive outside the womb, and (7) at birth.

I will talk about these in the chronological order in which they occur during human development.

---

[i] http://www.ipscell.com/2010/12/scientific-proof-for-the-dc-court-of-appeals-that-life-begins-at-conception-not-by-a-long-shot/

Before conception

The idea that life could begin before conception may seem counterintuitive at first, but let me explain. Most of the time for a human embryo to start growing, a sperm has to fertilize the egg forming a zygote, which then begins dividing. However, sometimes, an egg spontaneously starts the process of development on its own in an event termed "parthenogenesis" (Greek for "virgin birth").

Parthenogenesis occurs widely throughout life forms on Earth, but as far as I know it has not been proven to have naturally occurred in humans leading to an actual birth. Even so, given the number of people who have ever lived on Earth, it is possible that it has happened even if it has not been documented. It can also be stimulated in a lab in many species of oocytes including those of humans.

Parthenogenesis could theoretically produce a normal human female. So in theory, a human egg has the potential to create a living human being, although research to date suggests that human parthenogenic development (while readily activated in human eggs) does not proceed very often much beyond blastocyst formation and only rarely even makes it to that stage.[ii] Technological tweaks could make human parthenogenic babies quite possible, however.

Therefore, one might argue that a human egg is a living human being because of this *potential* for human parthenogenic development if one defines an entity as "human life" based on the potentiality to form a human being.

To me, this seems like a stretch, but keep it in mind as we go forward with our discussion considering the importance and limitations of potentiality. As a side note, it is also worth mentioning that parthenogenic stem cells have been produced and differentiated in a very similar manner to embryonic stem cells, for example to heart cells that might have useful clinical applications [1].

[ii]http://www.ncbi.nlm.nih.gov/pubmed/17706204

Conception

The case for human life beginning at conception is fairly straightforward, which is appealing in a way. It is undeniable that the first step (barring parthenogenesis discussed above or other artificial means discussed below) that needs to be taken to end up with a living, breathing human being is conception. However, the case against conception is that a fertilized human egg is not by any stretch of the imagination an actual human being.

The fertilized egg, also known as a zygote, has the potential to sometimes make a human being, but often it does not. From my perspective, a fertilized egg is not a person. It is instead very much like a seed. I find this analogy helpful so I want to build on it.

Imagine a redwood forest and a seed has just flitted down from a cone. A single mature redwood reportedly[iii] can make up to ten million seeds a year, a startling high number. Any individual single redwood seed has a chance to make a tree, but a very low chance. Clearly mature redwoods do not each produce ten million new actual trees every year.

Even if that seed has the potential to become a redwood tree over a period of years by growing billions or trillions of times in mass and developing leaves and other specialized structures, it does not mean that that seed *is* a tree. In fact the odds are very much against that seed ever becoming a living tree. First it has to implant in the ground, send out roots, and so forth.

One critical concept here is that potential does not mean equal. A seed can become a tree, but a seed is not a tree. They are different. A fertilized human egg can under just the right circumstances become a human being, but that potential does not equate the fertilized egg with a human being. The early human embryo has to survive, implant in the uterus, grow trillions of times in size, etc.

Thus, for me personally, conception is not when human life begins, but again that is not some universal "right" answer that I expect others to necessarily believe.

[iii]http://www.flowersociety.org/Redwood-profile.htm

A second important concept is that having a unique genetic identity does not make a cell or group of cells a human being. Proponents of the idea that life begins at conception also sometimes argue that since the zygote has its own genetic makeup that is distinct from the sperm and egg that it is therefore a human being. However, just as that redwood seed has a unique set of DNA different from its "parental" trees and yet is not itself a tree, a human zygote is not a human.

If unique genetic makeup were enough to define something as a human being then cancers would be their own human beings as their DNA is distinct from the person in which they form. Even the wart on my great-aunt's nose might be a human being if one buys the argument that a unique genetic identity defines something as a human being since warts can have unique elements of DNA.

Implantation

In human and other mammalian development, implantation is a key event. Implantation is the step in mammalian development when the hitherto free-floating embryo moving down the fallopian tube binds to a spot on uterus and starts connecting with the uterine tissues. Ultimately this is the only way an embryo can thrive via stimulating development of the placenta and a blood supply to the embryo.

In humans implantation occurs around 2 weeks after conception. I am not sure if human life begins at implantation, but I can see the appeal of this idea. Human implantation is very much like a seed sprouting into the ground. Certainly implantation must occur for the ultimate creation of a human being as no embryo can survive without becoming attached to the uterus. On the other hand, the embryo does not somehow directly change its intrinsic nature to become more human due to implantation.

Heart beat as the start?

Other folks believe that a human being truly begins when it has a heart beat. Indeed in North Dakota a law was just passed in March of 2013 and signed into law by the Governor of that state here in the US based on this idea. The law bans abortions based on a key timepoint of the appearance of a detectable fetal heartbeat (around 12 weeks of gestation),[iv] suggesting those lawmakers' sense that that is when a human being has started. A beating human heart can be a strong symbol of life, but whether this event qualifies as the start of the life of a human being is unclear to me.

Human brain activity as the beginning?

Another notion is that a human being "starts" its existence as a full, independent human when the developing brain starts functioning like that of a human. There is some debate about when this happens, but at the earliest it would seem to start in the 2nd trimester. Earlier than that a human brain can fire off random neuron activity, but from all evidence that I have seen, the early human fetal brain's electrical activity is nothing like the activity related to thoughts that is so distinctive in living, breathing human beings. It is more akin to chaotic electrical activity. Interestingly, even a dish of human neurons in the lab can produce measurable electrical activity. What we are talking about here as a defining point of the start of a human being is quite different: brain activity more similar to human thought. To me this brain-based definition is interesting, but very unclear. It lacks a clear starting point, more likely being something that gradually starts to become apparent and differs somewhat in every fetus.

Survival outside the womb

With advances in medical technology, the date at which a human fetus can survive outside the womb has gotten earlier over the years. With rare exceptions, the earliest such gestational date is 23 weeks of age, which is quite remarkable. Usually such fetuses do not survive, but sometimes they do. Even when they do survive, such "preemies" often are extremely ill for years and are at higher risk for numerous health problems as adults.

[iv]http://www.reuters.com/article/2013/03/26/us-usa-abortion-northdakota-idUSBRE92P0UA20130326

The notion that independent survival ability is the definition of the start of human life was the most common answer in the poll I did (which admittedly was far from scientific) on my blog.[v] I can see the appeal of this definition, but what makes it less than ideal is that this point of independent survival will be different for every fetus. It is a somewhat nebulous standard.

At birth

The appeal of this idea is that birth is such a well-defined event and is indisputably the time when a mother and the fetus/baby become separated. The baby starts breathing and crying. The baby will begin truly eating after this as well. She or he receives her or his own name and this is the time the baby is formally and legally recognized as a separate human being. The birth certificate is filled out.

As much as this definition is appealing and has a definite logic to it, to me personally, it seems a bit late. If for whatever reason labor starts weeks or even more than a month earlier than it would have otherwise, almost always this late fetus will survive. In this hypothetical scenario, is the fetus not a human until it formally separates from the mother even though it is essentially completely developed and can function independently if need be? These are tough questions.

Overview of ideas about when a living human being begins

Cultures around the world have many different answers about the start of life. For me a fertilized egg is not a human being. One's beliefs about when human life begins are certainly quite strongly influenced by one's parents, religion, cultural background, and other specific factors in one's life. Again, I do not believe that science or medicine have particularly definitive answers to this very challenging question.

---

[v]http://www.ipscell.com/2011/05/when-does-life-begin-our-poll-results/

Emerging Ethical Debates in the Stem Cell Field

While the embryonic stem cell debate continues perhaps a bit less intensely since the US Federal Court ruling definitively allowing federal funding of the research, stem cell-related technologies have in recent years raised other major ethical challenges.

Whereas the embryonic stem cell debate has been about, depending on one's perspective, ending (via using a blastocyst) or saving (via creating embryonic stem cell lines that can be used as medicines) human lives, emerging stem cell technologies raise different ethical questions. These dilemmas relate instead to use technology to create or change human beings.

While the possibility of a human, rather than God or nature, creating another human being and the dangers this could entail have been discussed for centuries (arguably most masterfully captured in Mary Shelley's *Frankenstein*), today's stem cell and reproductive technologies make the construction of such a human-made human or human-changed human far more realistic and I believe imminent (as in the next few decades). As a result, it is relatively more urgent now to address how society should deal with such a potential future reality for humanity at practical, legal, and ethical levels.

IVF: "Cure" for Infertility, But Also Gateway Technology for Questionable Practices?

In vitro fertilization (IVF) is a technique whereby infertile human couples can sometimes still produce healthy children.

How does IVF work?

In IVF, sperm and oocytes (i.e. human eggs, sometimes donated from another woman if the hopeful mother-to-be is infertile) are mixed in a dish in a lab, where fertilization can occur in vitro instead of inside of a woman. The goal is to help infertile couples become parents, which is admirable, but unfortunately IVF also is the gateway technology for many ethically questionable applications that could lead to the creation of genetically modified human beings.

The first goal of IVF is to create blastocyst stage embryos. Typically, many more such embryos are produced than are needed for attempts at pregnancy during which the embryos are implanted into the womb. Hundreds of thousands of such "leftover" blastocyst embryos remain frozen in liquid nitrogen around the world. Thousands are discarded each year. A few are used to make human embryonic stem cell lines.

IVF falls into a category of medicine called "assisted reproduction", which can also include injection of sperm or sperm nuclei into oocytes in the case of infertile men with sperm that are not normally motile or have other problems.

IVF has created children with 3 genetic parents

Many people may not realize that IVF technology has already been tweaked to create genetically modified human beings.

Yes, genetically modified humans already exist.

How did this happen?

Researchers and clinics in the assisted reproduction field have not been governed by strict laws in terms of what they can or cannot do via IVF. While lack of regulation has promoted "innovation" in IVF, in retrospect it appears that some risks related to IVF were underestimated and reproductive medicine should have been better regulated. More broadly, I contend that while people point to IVF as an example of the benefit of deregulation, current evidence suggests significant problems with that historical and philosophical narrative.

The ultimate goal of IVF clinics and doctors is to have a high success rate of producing children for their clients, infertile couples, so sometimes they have pushed the technology to the limit and their behavior has raised ethical questions.

IVF clinics at times in the past tried to "rescue" a woman's oocytes by infusing them with parts of a younger woman's oocytes. To this end, they injected the less-than-ideal oocyte of one woman with the oocyte cytoplasm of another woman to try to "rescue" the somewhat faulty oocyte. These hybrid oocytes are genetically distinct from either woman because they contain DNA from two women.

You might be saying to yourself something like, "but wait, the DNA is in the nucleus and you are saying cytoplasm was transferred so why are these new hybrid oocytes genetically modified?"

As it turns out all people have two kinds of DNA: nuclear and mitochondrial DNA. The latter is stored exclusively in the cytoplasm by cells and is always maternally inherited because sperm have no cytoplasm. Every one of us only gets our mitochondrial DNA (mtDNA) from our mothers.

Hybrid oocytes produced by cytoplasm transfer contain the genomic nuclear DNA of one woman, but the mtDNA of two women in the mixed cytoplasm of the hybrid. Such hybrid oocytes were reportedly fertilized and used to create actual people in the past.[vi]

However, the FDA has tried to stop the practice and has since not approved it. Whether non-compliant oocyte cytoplasmic transfer rescue still occurs in some IVF clinics in the US is unknown but possible. IVF clinics around the world may also be doing the same thing.

The reason the FDA tried to put a stop to the practice here in the US was that there were signs that the procedure had a higher rate of producing genetically abnormal children. These kids had chromosomal abnormalities presumably due to the manipulations of the oocytes. The process also raises significant, unresolved ethical issues since these children would have 3 genetic parents: two mtDNA moms one of which would also be a nuclear DNA mother, and a nuclear DNA dad.

Creating More Genetically Modified Humans to Potentially Treat Mitochondrial Diseases: Is It Worth the Risk?

Surprisingly, despite the troubling issues surrounding oocyte cytoplasmic transfer, some scientists today are advocating for even more dramatic oocyte-based artificial reproductive technologies.

There is a push by some today to allow for creation of genetically modified humans on several fronts. Going well-beyond cytoplasm transfer, some scientists are arguing for oocyte nuclear transfer technology to be allowed by the FDA to create actual new human beings.

[vi]http://www.fda.gov/OHRMS/DOCKETS/ac/02/slides/3855s1-05.pdf

In oocyte nuclear transfer, a whole egg nucleus is put into an entirely new oocyte cytoplasm, similar to what happens during cloning except using an egg nucleus instead of a somatic nucleus. A related reproductive technology called "spindle transfer", which does not transfer the whole nucleus, but just the chromosomes from one oocyte to another, is also being promoted.

Researchers in the US have published on these methods including in human cells as well as actual living, non-human primates [2, 3]. Some researchers want to now do this in humans.[vii] This proposed form of assisted reproduction would produce genetically modified human beings (two moms and one dad) and for that reason some are opposed to it, although Arthur Caplan, a prominent ethicist, stated at one time that he believes it is worth the risk.[viii] I have strong reservations about it.

How would this work to possibly address mitochondrial disorders?

The process is outlined in Figure 12.1. As mentioned above, human beings all have two kinds of DNA: nuclear and mitochondrial. In all cells the mtDNA, which is functional and important, is strictly cytoplasmic. Faulty mtDNA can lead to a host of health problems. As a result, researchers have proposed an assisted reproduction technology that would potentially address mtDNA diseases via oocyte nuclear transfer.

The scientists put forth the idea of creating an oocyte that has the nuclear DNA of the mother-to-be (who has faulty mtDNA) but has the mtDNA of another woman (let us call her "Ms. A") who has healthy mtDNA. The first step to create this hybrid oocyte is taking the nucleus of the mother-to-be's oocyte out of her oocyte, a process called enucleation. The oocyte of Ms. A would also have its nucleus removed via enucleation. Then, the researchers would take the mother-to-be's oocyte nucleus and put it inside Ms. A's enucleated oocyte, which contains normal mtDNA. In other words, they would do nuclear transfer. Alternatively, they would do spindle transfer (chromosomes, but not the whole nucleus) from one oocyte to another to avoid the disease prone mtDNA.

[vii]http://www.youtube.com/watch?v=o4K2TxOM-Ss&feature=youtu.be
[viii]http://vitals.nbcnews.com/_news/2012/10/24/14672441-ethicist-fixing-genes-using-cloning-technique-is-worth-the-ethical-risk?lite

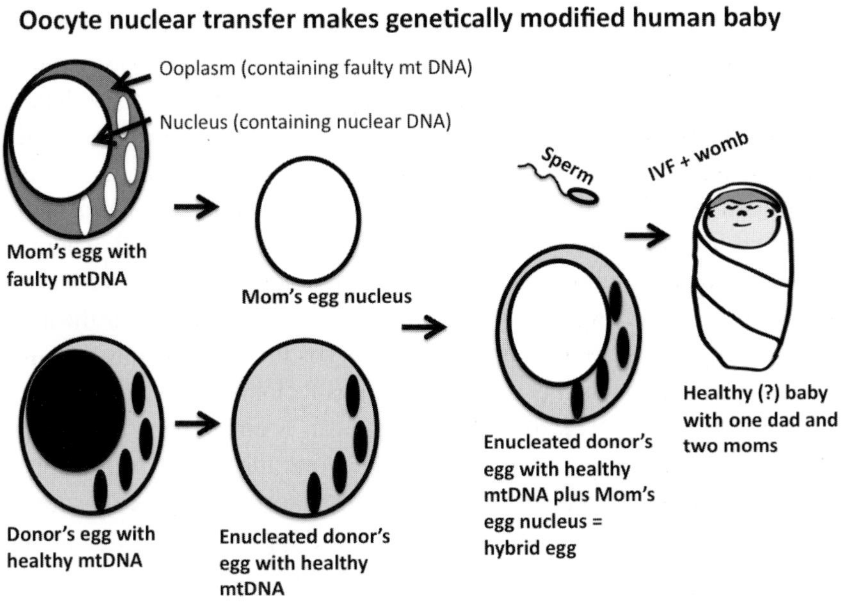

Oocyte nuclear transfer makes genetically modified human baby

Figure 12.1. How oocyte nuclear transfer would work to create a genetically modified human baby with 2 moms and hopefully no mtDNA disorder. Note that "ooplasm" simply refers to an oocyte's cytoplasm.

The modified oocyte that results from nuclear or spindle transfer would have the mother-to-be's nuclear DNA, but would have Ms. A's cytoplasm and hence her mtDNA. As a result, if fertilized and allowed to develop, the human being created using this method would have DNA from 3 people: 2 women (one woman's nuclear DNA and a different woman's mtDNA) and 1 man. Because Ms. A has normal mtDNA, the hope is that the person created from this technology would not have a mitochondrial disorder.

Scientists have demonstrated for human oocytes (strictly limited to the lab) [4, 5] and in primates going all the way through the creation of live offspring (seemingly normal) [6], that the technique can almost entirely eliminate faulty mtDNA.

However, there are three compelling arguments against allowing this technology to proceed on human beings.

First, there are the uncertain ethics of making genetically modified humans who can pass on the modifications to offspring. For example, a girl who was born of the proposed method would as an adult woman pass on to her daughters the mitochondrial DNA of another woman instead of her own.

Second, there is the ethics of potentially making very developmentally abnormal human babies because of the risks from this method. There is reason for concern about such risks because studies to date have shown that such bio-tinkering with oocytes can lead to defects in fertilization and sometimes lead to defects in early embryos produced in this way. As I will discuss next in the section on human cloning and somatic cell nuclear transfer (SCNT), the oocyte cytoplasm is collectively a powerful machine as well. What this mean is that beyond the new hybrid embryo having the DNA of 3 parents, we just do not know what the exposure of the patient's egg to another woman's egg cytoplasm might do to the patient's oocyte nuclear function and in turn to an actual person potentially created in this way.

Third, there is the risk of making genetic modifications of humans more culturally acceptable leading to eugenics.

Human Cloning and Its Technology

Human cloning is far more extreme than oocyte or nuclear transfer-based approaches to assisted human reproduction, but they share some methodological similarities such as modifying oocytes.

It is important to distinguish between two kinds of cloning. The first kind of cloning, the one that is the focus of this section, is technically called "reproductive cloning", which refers to making a second human being with the same DNA or genome as that of an already living human being.

The other main kind of cloning is called "therapeutic cloning" and it refers to producing a *cell line* that is genetically identical to an existing human being for either research or therapeutic purposes. These two kinds of cloning both depend on a process called somatic cell nuclear transfer (SCNT). A final, emerging possible kind of cloning would be based on iPS cell technology and depend on IVF.

Somatic Cell Nuclear Transfer (SCNT)

Somatic cell nuclear transfer (SCNT) is a nuclear juggling act that makes a new egg that contains instead of its own nucleus, the nucleus of another (non-stem, non-oocyte) somatic cell from a different human being.

In the first step of SCNT scientists enucleate a human oocyte. Remarkably, researchers are so skilled at enucleation these days that many of the resulting oocytes lacking nuclei remain intact and are not destroyed. They can remain viable for a short period of time with no nucleus, but will ultimately be ruined if they remain without a nucleus. Such enucleated oocytes are in essence a bag (cellular membrane) containing the gel of proteins and other factors (technically called "ooplasm" instead of cytoplasm in an oocyte, but I will continue to refer to it as "cytoplasm" here for consistency).

In the second step of SCNT, researchers remove the nucleus from a somatic cell. Again, skillful scientists can remove these somatic nuclei often without destroying them. In the case of the somatic cells, the rest of the cell can be discarded without interfering with the SCNT process.

In the third stage of SCNT, the somatic nucleus is injected into the enucleated oocyte. The injection uses a super thin micropipette that functions as a needle of just the right size. Its diameter is large enough so that the somatic nucleus can transit it without getting stuck or destroyed, but small enough such that it does not destroy the enucleated oocyte cytoplasm when inserted. Part of the reason that SCNT works at all is that oocytes are huge compared to the average cell, being at least ten times bigger.

In the fourth stage of SCNT, the new, now hybrid oocyte cell (oocyte membrane and cytoplasm possessing a somatic nucleus) adjusts to its new identity. What will dominate--the somatic nucleus or the oocyte components? Interestingly, in the subset of such hybrids that are still viable, almost always the cytoplasmic identity completely dominates.

After nuclear transfer, the somatic nucleus undergoes a process called "reprogramming" (akin to iPS cell formation) in which the oocyte cytoplasm makes the somatic nucleus now embedded within it change its epigenetic makeup so that it is nearly identical to that of an oocyte nucleus. Accordingly, at this stage the oocyte cytoplasm usually dominates and after "adjustment", its new somatic nucleus behaves almost precisely as an oocyte nucleus instead of a nucleus of the original cell (e.g. skin, blood, etc.) from which the somatic nucleus was taken. Note how similar cloning is to oocyte nuclear transfer mentioned in the previous section except here a somatic nucleus is transferred whereas in the other method an oocyte nucleus is transferred from one oocyte to a different one.

In the fifth stage of SCNT, the hybrid oocyte receives a shock and sometimes will start dividing. Remarkably, even in humans, a large fraction of shocked oocytes begin to divide and start to go through the first steps of embryogenesis.

It is at the sixth stage of SCNT that there is a fork in the road. Therapeutic and reproductive cloning follow separate paths here. In therapeutic cloning, the SCNT-produced embryo is cultured in a dish in the lab once it reaches the blastocyst stage to try to derive embryonic stem cell lines. In this way in theory any adult human could have an embryonic stem cell line made that has a matching genome to them via SCNT. There is hoped to be great therapeutic potential from such SCNT produced embryonic stem cell lines should they be proven to be normal, as they could be used potentially to make differentiated cells for autologous therapies.

In contrast, with reproductive cloning, the SCNT-produced early embryo is transferred to a host mother with the intent of producing a normal pregnancy and ultimately a living, cloned human organism. Who that mother would be, how she might be compensated, and who would pay for her medical care are questions that raise their own considerable ethical issues.

Both reproductive and therapeutic cloning have been successfully achieved in non-humans. For example, Dr. John Gurdon received the Nobel Prize[ix] for his work doing the first ever vertebrate reproductive cloning in frogs. Notably, I interviewed Dr. Gurdon for my blog and he clearly indicated that he is no fan of the idea of human reproductive cloning.[x]

[ix]http://www.nobelprize.org/nobel_prizes/medicine/laureates/2012/gurdon.html
[x]http://www.ipscell.com/2013/01/surprising-interviews-with-nobel-laureate-john-gurdon-and-bioethicist-art-caplan-on-human-cloning/

I also interviewed leading bioethicist Arthur Caplan on human cloning who discussed why it is such a nonsensical idea,[xi] a notion with which I totally agree. However, he and I disagree over the likelihood of human cloning becoming a reality. I think it is likely because of the rapid technological advances in the area as well as because of assorted human failings including hubris, a desire for power, and the quest for fame even amongst some scientists. Whether human reproductive cloning based on SCNT should be considered a stem cell-related procedure or not is up for debate.

One attempt at human therapeutic cloning led to the production of a genetically abnormal human embryonic stem cell line from SCNT that had more DNA than normal (it was triploid, having 3 sets of chromosomes instead the normal two, which is called a diploid state) [7]. A more recent paper reported successful human therapeutic cloning. Some concerns and questions remain about this paper at this time due to a number of errors in the manuscript, but my feeling at this time is that the process was successful.[xii]

I believe that human reproductive cloning will be successfully achieved in the next couple decades.

Why would this be a bad thing?

I am opposed to human cloning for many reasons. The most critical factor for me that raises red flags is the very real possibility that it might take 100 or more tries to get a single human clone that develops apparently normally.

What happens to the other 99 possibly malformed humans?

Another important reason for opposition is the fact that the clone (as well as any developmentally malformed semi-humans created during the process) would have no legal parents and an uncertain legal standing that could spark abuses. Even clones that appear normal as children could end up aging more rapidly than normal or having a very high incidence of cancer that only manifests later.

[xi]http://www.ipscell.com/2013/01/guest-post-by-art-caplan-on-human-reproductive-cloning/
[xii]http://www.ipscell.com/2013/05/human-cloning-cell-paper-under-investigation-some-perspectives/

How iPS Cell-Based Human Cloning Could Work

Beyond SCNT, iPS cell technology could also theoretically be used to clone human beings, but many questions remain.

Recall that iPS cells in principle can be made from any human being's somatic, non-stem cells. Much the same as embryonic stem cells, iPS cells can differentiate into any cell type in the body, including the gametes: eggs (oocytes) and sperm. Therefore, remarkably, iPS cell technology can in theory make sperm from women and eggs from men (Figure 12.2), opening the door to a possible unique form of reproductive cloning.

What this means is that in theory a woman alone can have cloned children derived from her natural eggs and fertilized with her own iPS cell-derived sperm that fertilize the eggs by IVF. Much the same, one man alone could in principle have children via his own natural sperm, which would be used to fertilize his iPS cell-derived eggs via IVF.

Further, two men could have a baby using one's sperm and eggs produced via iPS cell technology from the other man. Alternatively, two women could have children via one's eggs and the other's iPS cell-derived sperm. In any of these scenarios, no natural sperm or eggs may even be necessary since all gametes could be made from iPS cells.

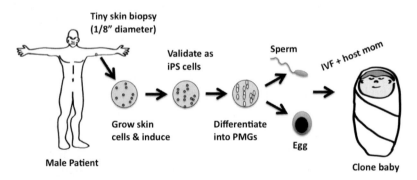

Figure 12.2. How a clone baby could theoretically be made using iPS cell technology. In theory with a male customer, either his own natural sperm or his iPS cell-derived sperm could be used. For a woman customer, her own eggs or her iPS cell-produced eggs could be utilized. For production of either iPS cell-based eggs or sperm, the likely first step needed is in vitro differentiation of the iPS cells into primordial germ cells (PMGs). Assuming the technology works to get to the fertilization point via IVF and the embryo develops, would the method create healthy babies? Nobody knows.

While scientists have derived sperm and eggs from skin cells using iPS cell technology and created mice in this way [8, 9], whether it would work in humans remains unknown. Even if the technology "works", would the humans created be "normal"? The only possible way to know is to try it out, which I think is a terrible idea, but nonetheless one that I expect will happen in the future despite ethical concerns.

Another possible approach to clone a human using iPS cells is to try using tricks developed in the mouse genetics field to directly use the iPS cells to fulfill the role of the ICM (Inner Cell Mass) cells.

If the technological issues could be worked out, another important question is whether iPS cell-based reproductive cloning is ethical. Many of the same ethical concern arise here as apply to SCNT-based cloning. Who would be the legal parents of iPS cell produced human clones? What happens if abnormal humans are produced in this way during the attempts to try out the technology? Who would be responsible for them? No one at this time has good answers to these important questions.

Phony Clone

Already, some have falsely claimed to have produced cloned human beings. In 2002, a religious group called the Räelian Movement announced that they had cloned a baby girl, Eve, leading to a media frenzy across the globe.[xiii] One of my stem cell policy mentors, Bernard Siegel, who is now the Executive Director of the Genetics Policy Institute, stepped in to address the situation and sought a guardian for Eve. He also exposed the bogus nature of the Räelians' cloning claim. However, today it seems we are dramatically closer to human cloning becoming a reality and one possible route, although certainly not the only one, to this dubious future would be through stem cell technology. When will that first real human clone will be produced and with what ethical costs and repercussions for humanity?

[xiii]http://www.nytimes.com/2002/12/28/us/group-says-human-clone-was-born-to-an-american.html

The Ethical Complexities of Human Egg Procurement

Some of the technologies discussed earlier depend on a source of human eggs. Human eggs are not something you can buy in cartons at the grocery store, but where do they come from exactly? Human eggs are obtained from women who must go through a complicated, invasive medical procedure that has risks (more on that below).

The sourcing of human eggs is a complicated ethical and legal issue of its own. Surprisingly, there are few state laws in the US, no definitive federal regulations in the US, and relatively few laws around the world concerning human egg donation specifically for stem cell research.

In 2009, New York became the first and only state in the US to permit compensation for eggs for stem cell research, based on specific ethical and legal guidelines [10]. Today in 2013, a California bill seeks to compensate women for the process of egg donation for research.[xiv] It may come as a surprise to many readers that the current law in California, based on a 2006 bill that was passed, states that women cannot be compensated beyond any direct expenses incurred from the egg donation process itself.

To obtain human eggs, women donors are needed. Each donor is compensated approximately $5,000-$10,000 in the US for her time and the "burden" of the ordeal. In other countries the compensation for this burden is considerably less than that in the US.

What is involved in egg donation?

The donors go through an invasive medical process that is at least a month long. It involves daily hormone injections that stimulate multiple ovulations to get more eggs, transvaginal ultrasounds, and blood tests. Ultimately the eggs produced must be retrieved from inside the woman, which can be painful. There are also medical risks:

> "Complications of oocyte donation range from bloating and mood swings to ovarian hyperstimulation syndrome, which can cause kidney damage and conditions necessitating ovary removal, or potentially some forms of cancer. Although

---

[xiv]http://www.sacbee.com/2013/03/10/5250417/california-bill-seeks-pay-for.html

serious complications are generally thought to be very rare,
the medical literature reflects uncertainty as to the frequency
and severity of these occurrences" [10].

The ordeal that the woman donor must go through is in fact a medical procedure and hence human subjects regulations apply. What this means it that those in charge of the egg donation process must technically have an IRB and state and federal approval for human subjects research, but sometimes they do not follow these rules.

Interestingly, egg donation is an area that both some liberals and conservatives can agree to oppose on ethical grounds. Certain liberals oppose egg donation on the grounds that it violates a woman's autonomy and is for that reason unethical. Some conservatives are opponents of egg donation because of the possibility that the eggs may be used to create embryos that might be destroyed to make embryonic stem cell lines, which they consider unethical. Other important ethical considerations include undue inducement/loss of autonomy and commodification of human eggs [10].

An ISSCR committee published a position statement on the procurement of human eggs for stem cell research in 2013 [11]. In that paper the committee pointed out the research needs for human eggs, and they stress that there is a shortage:

"Assuming that human embryonic stem cell research,
and research into infertility and mitochondrial disease, is
thought desirable, it is clear that there is a shortage of
human eggs for use in research and that many more eggs
will be needed."

The ISSCR committee presented nine conclusions that I have briefly summarized: (1) paying women for providing eggs (not for the eggs themselves) for research is ethically justifiable, (2) efforts should be made to avoid such payments becoming an inducement that could cross the line to "egg selling", (3) given the complex socioeconomic diversity of the world, the ISSCR is not in a position to specify payment amounts, but they argue for payments being capped, (4) centers that collect eggs should publish data on the process, (5) independent ethics committees are needed to ensure informed consent, (6) it is important to separate fertility treatment (i.e. involving women as patients) from recruited egg donors for research, (7) stem cell researchers have a responsibility to verify the ethical nature of the egg sourcing related to their work, (8) cross-border trade in eggs needs to be actively blocked to the extent possible, and (9) there needs to be more discussion at an international level over the issues surrounding egg donation.

I largely agree with the 9 conclusions of the ISSCR, but I am perhaps more directly and openly concerned about whether some so-called "research" uses of human eggs are ethically questionable. As you read earlier, I am also not particularly enthusiastic about tinkering with human development to try to address mitochondrial diseases and potentially create human babies with even more serious problems.

Summary

The ethical issues surrounding stem cells are complex and raise questions that have no easy, black-and-white answers. In my opinion, the most essential objective moving forward is to continue discussing these issues and avoid doing medical procedures based on dramatic technological leaps that may create genetically altered (and potentially developmentally abnormal) human beings before we have a meaningful ethical framework to determine whether or not these practices should be allowed to occur.

References

1. Didie, M, et al. (2013) Parthenogenetic stem cells for tissue-engineered heart repair. *The Journal of clinical investigation*.
2. Paull, D, et al. (2012) Nuclear genome transfer in human oocytes eliminates mitochondrial DNA variants. *Nature*. **493**:7434:632-7.
3. Tachibana, M, et al. (2013) Towards germline gene therapy of inherited mitochondrial diseases. *Nature*. **493**:7434:627-31.
4. Paull, D, et al. (2012) Nuclear genome transfer in human oocytes eliminates mitochondrial DNA variants. *Nature*.
5. Craven, L, et al. (2010) Pronuclear transfer in human embryos to prevent transmission of mitochondrial DNA disease. *Nature*. **465**:7294:82-5.

6. Tachibana, M, et al. (2009) Mitochondrial gene replacement in primate offspring and embryonic stem cells. *Nature.* **461**:7262:367-72.
7. Noggle, S, et al. (2011) Human oocytes reprogram somatic cells to a pluripotent state. *Nature.* **478**:7367:70-5.
8. Hayashi, K, et al. (2012) Offspring from oocytes derived from in vitro primordial germ cell-like cells in mice. *Science.* **338**:6109:971-5.
9. Hayashi, K, et al. (2011) Reconstitution of the mouse germ cell specification pathway in culture by pluripotent stem cells. *Cell.* **146**:4:519-32.
10. Roxland, BE (2012) New York State's landmark policies on oversight and compensation for egg donation to stem cell research. *Regenerative medicine.* **7**:3:397-408.
11. Haimes, E, et al. (2013) Position statement on the provision and procurement of human eggs for stem cell research. *Cell Stem Cell.* **12**:3:285-91.

Chapter 13

Getting Your Stem Cell Geek On

Stem cell technology is in some cases so cutting-edge that it inspires all kinds of cool, but geeky ideas. Some of these concepts are more in the realm of fiction such as sci-fi, while others are quite real or look to soon become part of a new reality. **We have reached a point where stem cell non-fiction is more interesting than the fiction.** Both can be quite fascinating and even entertaining, although the fictional stem cell beliefs sometimes do get in the way of progress.

Certain realities of the stem cell field are remarkably paradoxical, while many myths and urban legends are based on stem cells as well. Stem cells are increasingly becoming a part of pop culture and have appeared in quite a number of recent movies. For example, I wrote a blog piece[i] on actress Emma Stone talking about stem cells in the most recent *SpiderMan* movie. In advance of the movie she went to an actual research lab and learned about stem cells. She seemed very excited about stem cells and the cells played a role in that movie as well.

As stem cell therapies advance as potential medicines, more and more people are getting enthralled with and involved in stem cell-based ventures. Some are taking the next step to consider stem cell procedures or have actually already gotten them.

In this chapter, I guide you through some of the most creative and mindboggling stem cell-related inspirations, real or imagined. I also fill you in some of the darkest secrets of the stem cell field.

---

[i]http://www.ipscell.com/2012/06/emma-stone-dishes-on-spiderman-and-stem-cells-very-cool/

Whether genuine or invented, these stem cell mind-bogglers entertain, amuse, and even stimulate the mind. I will start by discussing what I think are some especially awesome and yes, perhaps even somewhat geeky stem cell inspirations.

Cool Stem Cell Ideas

Stem cells have entered mainstream culture. They are routinely mentioned in movies and TV shows. They are so eye-popping and cutting edge that everyday Americans are now frequently talking about them. On a recent trip to give a talk at the UCLA Stem Cell Center in 2013 I found an ad for stem cell procedures in the inflight magazine. In this section I discuss some of the more odd, but fun areas of potential stem cell research applications.

Even if you are not a geek, get your stem cell geek on just for the moment and have some fun with these ideas!

Organ replacement: The stem cell human body shop?

One area of stem cell research that seems like sci-fi, but is on track to become a reality in the next decade or two is organ replacement. One common reason why people die prematurely is that one of their critical organs fails. Most of the rest of the body could be healthy and yet the person dies. It could be their heart, kidneys, lungs, or liver that fails.

Of course serious damage to other organs from injury or illness such as the pancreas may not be immediately fatal, but can lead to lifelong problems and ultimately indirectly to premature death such as in some diabetics. In the future when we face organ failure instead of dying or facing a life of medical problems, we may be able to make a new organ via stem cells to replace the old one.

It is not just internal organs, but also other body parts that may be replaced in the future via stem cells. The range of external body part replacements being investigated by stem cell researchers and bioengineers is a laundry list that might include some surprises for you: skin, fingers, toes, entire limbs, breasts, hair, and genitals.

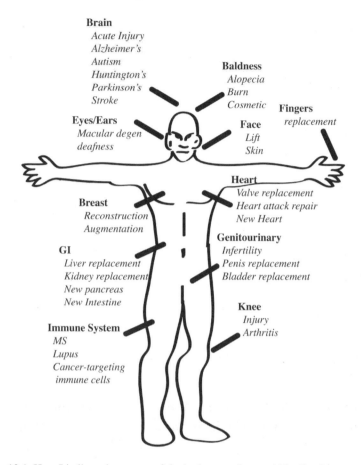

Figure 13.1. Here I indicate just some of the body parts that could be fixed, augmented or replaced via stem cells.

For genital replacement, an NBC journalist interviewed me about stem cells in a general sense and she ended up publishing an article quoting me. I did not even know the story was focused in part on penis replacement until it was published.[ii] As surprising as this application of stem cells may sound, this type of medical application is important. For example, soldiers can have devastating genital injuries on the battlefield.

[ii]http://www.nbcnews.com/id/48976348/ns/health-mens_health/#.UUuAKo6bFVQ

Lessons from "lower" organisms about regeneration

How would organ or body part replacement work?

Surprisingly, some of the best lessons in this regard come from so-called "lower" organisms, which paradoxically have far more regenerative power than humans.

I confess.

I am jealous of frogs, lizards, salamanders and even simple worms.

Why?

I envy them because of their cellular and tissue transdifferentiation potential. Their body parts have the remarkable ability to transform or regrow.

At best humans can regrow the tip of their finger if it gets cut off or part of our liver if we drink too much on a regular basis or get hepatitis.

There was an article recently in the journal *Nature Communications* about the striking regenerative capacity of salamanders [1]. They can regrow many different body parts including stunningly, the lens of their eyes. Researchers showed that this lens regeneration function, which is a stem cell-dependent function, surprisingly does not seem to diminish with age or with repeated loss of the same tissue structure.

If you are a human, this amphibian retention of regeneration capacity with age is not much consolation since we start out even as kids without much of any ability to regenerate organs anyway. But think again. The studies on so-called "lower" organisms that have near complete regenerative capacity nonetheless may someday provide insight into how to unlock the potential ability of humans to regenerate tissues including limbs, digits and other human body parts. However, even if we humans never can regrow limbs or even digits, studies on creatures like lizards and salamanders (which when it comes to regeneration are really the "higher" organisms) may very well provide clues for stem cell-based regenerative medicine for us humans.

We have a lot to learn still and some of it from creatures that seem far removed from us humans. Some of these critters, upon tissue damage such as the loss of a limb, form an intriguing structure called a blastema.

What is a blastema?

A blastema is a specialized regenerative structure that either contains stem cells to start with or gets a fresh supply of stem cells from in vivo cellular reprogramming. As far as we know, humans do not make blastemas if injured as adults, which is likely why we cannot regenerate tissues. Learning more about the blastema of other animals could teach us how to unlock human regeneration.

Since humans apparently do not have blastema or the equivalent of these kind of regenerative centers, our best bet for replacing body parts comes from stem cell-based laboratory bioengineering of organs.

However, some organisms go well beyond regrowing a limb and exhibit far more robust regeneration capacity. For example, when cut into small pieces, the simple planarian worm can regenerate entire new worms from many of the small pieces, some as small as 1/279th of the original body mass. How it achieves this wondrous regeneration remains unknown, but appears to depend on the fact that about one in six of the total cells in the mature planarian worm is a cell called a "neoblast" that is akin to an embryonic stem cell in terms of its potency.

It is thought that adult humans lack such pluripotent cells because the cells would pose too high a risk of cancer. For example, when humans get teratoma tumors or even teratocarcinoma (a malignant form of teratoma), it is thought to be caused by residual pluripotent stem cells accidentally leftover in the body from embryonic development.

De-extinction and extinction prevention

De-extinction

Various teams of scientists around the world are interested in using stem cell technology combined with genomics to bring back various creatures from the dead. There was even an entire scientific conference in 2013 devoted to the topic of de-extinction.[iii]

In the movies, such efforts included the case of dinosaurs in *Jurassic Park*, but lately two other extinct creatures have been seriously discussed

---

[iii]http://www.ted.com/tedx/events/7650

as potential candidates for de-extinction via stem cell technology: wooly mammoths and Neanderthals. In the latter case, some scientists are talking about how one would hypothetically go about cloning Neanderthals back into existence.[iv]

In regards to wooly mammoths, reportedly scientists have already started that project.[v] The wooly mammoth project is a team effort of Russian scientists and South Korean stem cell researcher, Hwang Woo-suk. Some may remember Woo-suk for being involved in many controversies surrounding human cloning [2].

Whether any of these geeky bring-cool-creatures-back-to-life efforts will succeed in the future is anybody's guess. However, as stem cell technology continues to advance along with other powerful methods like next generation genome sequencing and synthetic life, the future of biomedical research in this area should prove interesting.

Extinction prevention

Human beings are responsible for the extinction of many species and it seems like every day more species are threatened. Our activities as a society threaten some species via habit destruction and pollution. In addition poachers and other individuals are directly driving some species extinct. For hundreds of years, potential human-caused extinctions, once they occurred, were irrevocable.

Now, however, some scientists are trying to preserve endangered species in a creative way using stem cells. While de-extinction in theory is an option for species that are lost, a more proactive approach is to create an iPS cell bank that contains iPS cells from all endangered species. Not only could such a bank help with de-extinction efforts of recently lost species, but also it could be used prior to extinction to create cloned new individuals of an endangered species such as the rhino.[vi]

[iv]http://www.ipscell.com/2013/01/'adventurous'-woman-sought-to-carry-neanderthal-baby-candidate-for-dumbest-stem-cell-story-of-2013-already-pops-up-already/
[v]http://newsfeed.time.com/2012/03/14/the-woolly-mammoths-return-scientists-plan-to-clone-extinct-creature/
[vi]http://www.nature.com/news/2011/110904/full/news.2011.517.html

An important question of course is whether iPS cell-cloned animals would be healthy and fertile. Could this also dangerously make human reproductive cloning seem more acceptable to society?

Stem cell-produced meat: Show me the bacon!

Famine is a serious, global problem. Too many people including children go to bed hungry. Could this problem be solved by stem cell technology? Perhaps someday. One way that stem cell technology is already making a difference in the food industry is through widespread cloning of farm animals such as cows that each produce more meat than the average animal; however, many researchers do not believe that cattle are a means to help famine because they have a major negative impact on the environment.

What if one could create synthetic meat in a lab and make tons of it very cheaply? Some researchers have already started to explore the notion in the lab. They have started with the odd objectives of first making stem cell-produced bacon[vii] and burgers.[viii]

Not surprisingly, many questions remain including the safety and palatability of lab-grown meat as well as cost, but a few scientists are very seriously investigating this idea.

Zombie stem cells

One of the stranger developments in the field is the appearance of zombie stem cells.[ix] What exactly are zombie stem cells? It turns out that after we die that most of our cells stay still alive for a surprisingly long time. In fact, large populations of cells in a dead body remain alive for

---

[vii]http://www.mnn.com/green-tech/research-innovations/stories/scientists-grow-bacon-from-stem-cells
[viii]http://www.forbes.com/sites/michellemaisto/2012/02/22/stem-cell-burgers-coming-this-fall-are-you-ready-for-lab-to-table-eating/
[ix]http://www.ipscell.com/2012/06/tgif-the-good-bad-and-zombie-stem-cell-headlines-for-week-of-june-15/

weeks. This paradoxical post-death cellular survival includes stem cells.[x] Some scientists have even proposed the potential clinical use of zombie stem cells harvested weeks after death [3]. This notion may seem less odd when you consider that corpses are currently used as sources of other body parts for medical applications such as kidneys, lenses, and so forth, but typically in such applications the body parts must be isolated "fresh" immediately after death.

Stem cells in space

How would stem cells fare in space? What might be the effects of low gravity and cosmic radiation? Surprisingly, there have already been many NASA studies on stem cells. They found that space and changes in gravity alter the properties of stem cells in a variety of ways.[xi] Future experiments are already planned as well.[xii] My sense is that endogenous stem cells in astronauts are unlikely to be positively influenced by space. More likely, the longer human beings spend in space, the more probable it will become that they have stem cell dysfunction. Perhaps astronauts will age more rapidly in space.

Arguably one of the biggest hurdles to manned space flight in general, but particularly to other interesting places in the universe such as potentially habitable exoplanets is the huge amount of energy required to move human astronauts around in space due to our mass.

I have some interesting ideas about how to get around this problem including using stem cells, which have almost zero mass compared to adult astronauts. One notion is to send stem cells in the form of totipotent one-celled human zygotes and cells programmed to build a womb, in a frozen, protected form on the space journey. Once the ship arrives at its

[x]http://www.huffingtonpost.com/2012/06/13/stem-cells-corpses_n_1592935.html?ncid=edlinkusaolp00000003
[xi]http://www.nasa.gov/mission_pages/station/research/experiments/895.html
http://www.nasa.gov/mission_pages/station/research/experiments/494.html
http://www.nasa.gov/mission_pages/station/research/experiments/851.html
http://www.nasa.gov/centers/ames/news/releases/2010/10-23AR_prt.htm
[xii]http://www.newscientist.com/article/dn23220-stem-cells-aboard-spacex-will-seed-mice-back-on-earth.html

location, say a planet predicted to have large amounts of organic material, the ship utilizes those resources to grow an artificial womb from the stem cells and then triggers the development of the zygotes. Over a period of years, the astronauts would be literally grown on location from the stem cells.

Of course there are some issues such as the fact that the humans created at this other planet could never come back, but perhaps they could establish a colony there. After embryonic and fetal development, there is also the issue of who would take care of the infants and children. While it seems entirely feasible to have the ship's computer raise and educate them, it is less clear whether such children would be normal.

Interestingly, stem cells have played prominent roles in some sci-fi movies and series including *The Bourne Legacy* (stem cell-doped super spies), *The Amazing SpiderMan* (stem cell experiments mentioned), and *Battlestar Galactica* (hybrid fetal stem cells save the President on the show from cancer). While stem cells were only infrequently plot elements in *Star Trek*, a real life connection has been forged with the $5 million founding of the Roddenberry Stem Cell Center at UCSF.[xiii]

Myths and Urban Legends

The stem cell field has its share of myths and urban legends.

Certain people use myths and urban legends to advocate for or against specific ethical or moral precepts. I believe that dispelling these myths and legends will be helpful for you in understanding the stem cell field. Besides, some of them are fun and entertaining, while all no matter how frustrating are important to be aware of as a stem cell expert.

One might say that stem cell mythology can be traced back all the way to the Greek Titan Prometheus. Legend held that Prometheus, having angered Zeus, was cursed to have his liver eaten every day by a ferocious eagle, but his liver regenerated each time. Some believe this myth is based on real Greek knowledge of liver regeneration [4].

What are today's stem cell myths?

[xiii]http://gladstoneinstitutes.org/roddenberry

Myth #1: There are stem cells in Pepsi™

One of the most ridiculous stem cell urban legends is that the drink Pepsi has stem cells in it. Others have said that stem cells are used in the production of Pepsi. In turns out that both of these assertions are false. The Pepsi company works with another company on the developmental of new artificial flavorings and this company uses various cell lines in their work including one called HEK 293 (commonly called just "293" in the cell biology world). The HEK moniker is an acronym for "human embryonic kidney", but as it turns out even this is a misnomer as the cells were obtained from a *fetal* kidney.

While it is correct that the 293 line came from a single aborted fetus, these cells are not at all similar to embryonic stem cells. In addition, they do not appear to have any potency at all indicating they are not stem cells of any kind. In addition 293 cells are not actually in the Pepsi soft drink product that is sold and are only used in related research.

293 cells are a laboratory workhorse cell line with great flexibility. They are used for research every day in hundreds of labs around the world to study everything from cell and molecular biology to protein biochemistry. They have played a vital role in advancing biomedical research.

Myth #2: Stem cells, when eaten, are an aphrodisiac

So if you cannot drink stem cells in a soft drink, how about slurping them in your soup? In the Introduction to this book (see Figure I.3) I showed a picture of my stem cell alphabet soup. It turns out there is at least one other kind of stem cell soup, but a much more disturbing kind.

Stem cells are a hot topic all around the globe, but they are particularly scorching hot in certain countries such as the Philippines. There are an increasing number of news articles on stem cells and stem cell procedures out of news sources from the Philippines.

My white paper on stem cells for my Stem Cell Outreach Program for Education (SCOPE)[xiv] in Tagalog (the official language of the Philippines) is generating a great deal of interest there.

[xiv]http://www.ipscell.com/scope-global-stem-cell-outreach-program-for-education/

In the Philippines, dubious adult stem cell procedures are the rage. The government in March of 2013 announced a planned crackdown on dubious stem cell clinics.[xv]

I am sure there is great, legitimate stem cell research including clinical research in the Philippines and I have deep respect for the country and all Filipinos, but it seems that dubious stem cell procedures are as big a problem there as they are in the US and other places.

For example, we have the case of so-called Soup No. 7.

What is Soup No. 7?

In the Philippines there are various remedies for health that are called "soups" colloquially.

For example, there is Soup No. 5 made of bull testicles that is supposed to be an aphrodisiac.[xvi]

Now there is Soup No. 7.

I was unable to find a recipe, but it is a stem cell potion of sorts that Filipinos are strongly recommended **against** taking by doctors there as per this recent news item,[xvii] which included the following:

> "Leo Olarte, vice president and spokesman for the Philippine Medical Association (PMA), said bogus stem cell products now proliferate.
> "Products like soup number 7, which allegedly contain stem cells that can boost sexual appetite, are now being sold, but all these are fake and fraudulent," he said."

What does a stem cell soup have to do with sex? Not sure.

Not only are these soups unlikely to help anyone, but they could also be harmful. The article goes on to say:

> "Christian Emmanuel Mancao, of the Philippine Society for Stem Cell Medicine (PSSCM), said stem cells could

---

[xv]http://newsinfo.inquirer.net/382503/spas-salons-warned-on-stem-cell-therapy
[xvi]http://en.wikipedia.org/wiki/Soup_Number_Five
[xvii]http://www.abs-cbnnews.com/nation/metro-manila/02/28/13/doctors-warn-public-soup-no-7

not be turned into powder and put in vials because the body needs it alive in order to multiply and replace dead cells.

He said the stem cells must be injected into the body for it to be effective, and consumers must also ensure they use only products approved by the Food and Drug Administration (FDA)."

Stem cells are likely to only increase in hype around the world including both in the US and the Philippines as well as elsewhere. I believe the US has its own big problems with bogus stem cell procedures so I am by no means singling out the Philippines. I am an advocate for education and patient safety across the globe. Stem cell soup is something you should definitely pass on no matter what name or number it goes by or where it is sold. Have something delicious instead from the amazing offerings of Filipino cooking such as lechón.

Myth #3: Adult and autologous stem cells are by definition safe

One of the myths common in the stem cell world, propagated largely by non-compliant for-profit stem cell clinics, is that adult stem cells are by definition safe. They claim that adult stem cell procedures have basically zero risk. While adult stem cells are lower risk as a basis for treatments than other kinds of stem cells, there is no such thing as "no risk" when it comes to any medical treatment including adult stem cells.

Some patients have died.[xviii]

Another false claim is that an autologous stem cell procedure is by definition safe, when we know that some recipients of such procedures have had devastating side effects as discussed earlier in the book.

[xviii]http://www.cellmedicinesociety.org/home/news/latest/317-icms-announces-investigation-findings

Myth #4: iPS cells eliminate the need for embryonic stem cells

With the advent of iPS cells it was interesting to see that both stem cell advocates in general and opponents of embryonic stem cells could agree on one thing: iPS cells are very promising and powerful. However, the opponents of embryonic stem cells went a step further and promoted the myth that iPS cells immediately made embryonic stem cells unnecessary. We had barely gotten to know iPS cells and these folks were already proclaiming them as a godsend. To this day, seven years after the first mouse iPS cells were reported, we still do not know if iPS cells will ever replace embryonic stem cells. Interestingly, opponents of embryonic stem cell research are now increasingly showing opposition to iPS cells because they see them as unnatural and they might be used in cloning.[xix]

Myth #5: There is a conspiracy to kill adult stem cell therapies

I am admittedly an advocate of a relatively high degree of regulatory oversight of stem cell therapies by the FDA in the US and by similar regulatory agencies around the world. I believe this is necessary and appropriate as well as legally mandated in the US at least. However, I also advocate for some specific, logic reforms at the FDA as well (see Chapter 7).

Some non-compliant clinic advocates, fearing that access to their for-profit procedures is being hindered by the FDA, have created a myth that the FDA is in cahoots with "Big Pharma" to impede stem cell research. Their false logic goes that the FDA is in the pocket of big pharmaceutically companies that make their money off of traditional chemical "pill" drugs that somehow are threatened by new stem cell procedures.

[xix]http://www.ipscell.com/2013/05/why-the-extreme-religious-right-are-turning-against-ips-cells/

In all my years in the stem cell field I have never had any ties to big or small pharmaceutical or biotech companies (on some level I wish I did because that can speed the development of new therapies) so I feel I can speak independently to say there is no conspiracy. I see no evidence of this kind of situation and I believe that those who spread this myth do so as a way to try to discredit the FDA and to attack proponents of appropriate regulatory oversight.

Myth #6: Embryonic stem cells come from abortions

Embryonic stem cells have been a focal point of debates, what some would further call a war, in the stem cell arena. While the opponents of embryonic stem cells in the US have suffered a tremendous defeat with the definitive federal court ruling establishing federal funding of embryonic stem cell research as legal, I expect the fight will go on although perhaps with lower intensity.

One of the weapons used by the opponents of embryonic stem cells in their propaganda war against research in this area was to propagate the notion that embryonic stem cells come from abortions. This is false as embryonic stem cells are derived from early stage (100-cell) embryos only a few days old produced in labs by IVF, not from natural pregnancies.

Secrets

Secret clinic-patient confidentiality clauses

Within the for-profit stem cell field it is a fairly common practice for companies to require patients to sign confidentiality agreements as a condition for treatment. Therefore, any patient who will not sign is excluded and this introduces bias into the study, assuming the procedure is part of a study at all. In addition, often times the existence of the confidentiality agreement is itself agreed upon to be confidential as well. The confidentiality agreement itself becomes a secret.

It is notable that this kind of arrangement can exist with pharmaceutical companies as well when they conduct trials so it is not specific just to the non-compliant for-profit stem cell clinic area, but nonetheless such secrecy raises concerns for patient safety.

Additional contractual clauses can include restrictions on what patients may do in the event of negative outcomes or conflicts arising from their stem cell treatment. Such clauses, for example, may stipulate that patients may not sue their doctors or the clinic (although that generally does not hold up in court), but instead the parties must go into confidential arbitration in the event of conflict.

Secret patient websites

Another cloak and dagger element in the stem cell arena is the mostly hidden reality that patients and dubious clinics have secret websites. These websites are accessible by invitation-only and in theory serve as a place where patients can interact in a private, "safe" environment. Unfortunately, these websites also have as members fake patients as well as real patients who are paid advocates for specific clinics. As such, these sites often operate to promote more stem cell procedures and promulgate claims from clinics about safety and efficacy of stem cell procedures outside the domain where stem cell scientists and regulators can engage.

The cut-throat nature of the stem cell field

The stem cell field is not all one big happy family. There are cliques and different factions as well as some big egos all at play. Certain conflicts arise because of course some scientists wants to be the first to publish big discoveries and if they are not first, they might be angry with the person who is first. This may sound unprofessional or counterproductive, but competition is at the heart of all science and the stem cell field is not immune.

The cutthroat nature of the stem cell field manifests in very real ways that impact not just scientists, but also patients. In one sense, the fiercely competitive nature of the stem cell field is good because it drives discovery at a rapid pace. On the other hand, the intensity and strong feelings have negative repercussions including skewing review of papers and grants. In some instances, worthy grants and papers are killed by competitors for non-scientific reasons, a phenomenon I discuss in more detail in a satiric blog post.[xx]

Stem Cell Paradoxes

Most stem cell therapies will not transplant stem cells

An interesting paradox in the field of stem cell transplants exists: many stem cell transplants in the future will likely not contain actual stem cells. Instead, doctors will transplant patients with cells that are first differentiated in the lab from stem cells.

There are several distinct advantages of not using the stem cells themselves and instead using differentiated progeny of stem cells. First, differentiated cells are proven to generally have a far better safety profile in terms of the risk of tumor formation. Second, pre-differentiating the stem cells prior to transplant means you have a more homogeneous product.

However, there are also disadvantages to pre-differentiation. One of the most exciting aspects of stem cells is their potency, meaning the ability to form a variety of differentiated daughter cells. By pre-differentiating cells in the lab prior to transplant, you are sacrificing that potency.

Naïve stem cells directly transplanted are likely to respond to the body's cues more directly and by retaining potency may yield a better clinical result. For example, stem cells directly transplanted into the brain (as opposed to using neural cells pre-differentiated in the lab from those stem cells) may differentiate into many cell types that together make up a functional brain tissue including blood vessels needed for health. In contrast, just transplanting neurons or oligodendrocytes, another type of brain cell, has no potential to create a diverse tissue.

[xx]http://www.ipscell.com/2012/05/dirty-dozen-easy-steps-to-killing-a-paper-during-review-elephant-in-the-lab-series/

Transplantation of naïve stem cells may also yield higher engraftment, survival, and migration rates than using pre-differentiated cells. For any given disease or injury, doctors and scientists need to weigh the potential advantages and disadvantages of laboratory differentiation of stem cells prior to treatment.

At this time the dominant paradigm among researchers following FDA rules it to pre-differentiate stem cells prior to treatments, while interestingly at for-profit stem cell clinics, patients are treated essentially 100% of the time with undifferentiated stem cells.

Many stem cells are most similar to cancer cells

Before there were embryonic stem cells there were embryonal carcinoma cells (ECCs) isolated from mouse and human tumors. ECCs have many stem cell characteristics and research on ECCs provided the foundation for the first mouse embryonic stem cell studies that only came later.

The first stem cell treatment was not known for sure to depend on stem cells

Bone marrow transplantation was the first stem cell treatment and remains by far the one that has proven to be most successful. However, at the beginning of bone marrow transplant research, the teams studying it did not know for sure that it was a stem cell-based therapy.

"Adult" stem cell research does not always use only adult stem cells

As mentioned earlier in the book, people sometimes make the mistake of calling iPS cells and even at times fetal stem cells by the name "adult stem cells". As a result, therapies based on these stem cells are often mistakenly called "adult stem cell treatments". Umbilical cord blood stem cells from newborns are also technically wrongly termed "adult stem cells" by many people.

The main way that scientists measure pluripotency is a tumor assay

When scientists want to know just how "good" their embryonic stem cells and iPS cells are in terms of the cells' pluripotency, their standard test is the teratoma formation assay in immunodeficient mice. The teratoma assay is considered the gold standard, especially for human pluripotent stem cells. Researchers are working to develop additional pluripotency assays that do not involve teratoma [5].

Summary

Stem cells will continue to excite the scientist or even geek in all of us, whether they are discussed in the fictional or reality-based worlds we inhabit. I expect incarnations of stem cells in sci-fi will in some cases become part of fresh unexpected realities. New myths will emerge. All in all the stem cell field will continue to surprise and amaze.

References

1. Eguchi, G, et al. (2011) Regenerative capacity in newts is not altered by repeated regeneration and ageing. *Nature communications.* **2**:384.
2. Cyranoski, D (2009) Woo Suk Hwang convicted, but not of fraud. *Nature.* **461**:7268:1181.
3. Latil, M, et al. (2012) Skeletal muscle stem cells adopt a dormant cell state post mortem and retain regenerative capacity. *Nature communications.* **3**:903.
4. Taub, R (2004) Liver regeneration: from myth to mechanism. *Nature reviews. Molecular cell biology.* **5**:10:836-47.
5. Muller, FJ, et al. (2011) A bioinformatic assay for pluripotency in human cells. *Nature methods.* **8**:4:315-7.

Chapter 14

Conclusion: The Future of Stem Cells

It may be hard for us today to even conceive of just how many infectious diseases (now prevented by vaccines or cured with antibiotics) used to be not only both relatively common, but also almost uniformly fatal to people. I wonder if our grandchildren will feel the same way about organ replacement or other remarkable potential applications of stem cell-based regenerative and cellular medicine.

As with anything new, the potential benefits can seem endless, and the drawbacks are largely unknown. If we use caution and avoid the hype, we will minimize the risk of potential heartaches over the inevitable bumps in the road and sidestep outright landmines that potentially await the stem cell field as it moves forward. These kinds of hazards in a general sense are not unique to stem cells, but are simply a natural part of any medical revolution.

I am thrilled to be part of the cutting edge stem cell research going on, and in part it has motivated me to blog about this subject as well as write this book you are reading. Perhaps it also should not have surprised me that over the last two years many unlicensed, for-profit companies and their allies have reacted in a hostile way towards me. They do not like my positions promoting evidence-based medicine and my arguing for requirements for extensive safety data regarding the clinical use of specific stem cell procedures. They have even resorted to nasty personal attacks and threatened litigation. But as a researcher, father and potential future patient/recipient of these powerful cells, I will continue to publicly urge caution despite the price I pay for speaking my mind publicly. At the same time I will also talk about the many inspiring positives of the stem cell world too, of which there are many. Further, I encourage FDA reforms as well that will help more people.

Too often in the academic section of the stem cell field, people pussyfoot around the most important issues or do not even dare talk about them at all. My feeling is it is far more useful to have open discussions on controversial issues. We must engage in a dialogue (e.g. via this book) on such issues and doing so is worth the risk of upsetting some people. Hence in this book I have told you frankly my thoughts on the pressing stem cell issues of the day.

I can truly empathize with those people who have the intense range of negative and deeply scary emotions related to dealing with a life threatening or life changing medical condition. My own experience of being diagnosed with a very serious form of prostate cancer in 2009 put me in that position. Being in long-term remission rather than cured of prostate cancer, I can relate to uncertainty felt by many stem cell patients. Some people in that kind of situation may feel that they have little to lose and a lot of gain. It is not my place to convince them otherwise.

But at the same time, being a human guinea pig in a virtually uncontrolled, unmonitored setting and paying tens of thousands of dollars for a stem cell intervention that can only be termed "experimental" is not just going out on a limb, it is hanging onto a mighty thin stem at the end.

While I am not on some crusade to dissuade people from getting risky stem cell procedures, I do consider it part of my mission to voice concerns about the safety of certain stem cell procedures and encourage better training and education of providers. I also believe that noncompliant stem cell corporations threaten the entire stem cell field with their reckless behavior.

I urge people to exercise caution and to use common sense regarding their health, especially when it comes to using stem cells to treat medical conditions, whether life threatening or cosmetic in nature. Again, the potential is virtually unimaginable at this time. Talk to your doctors. Ask many questions and keep my Stem Cell Patient Bill of Rights (Chapter 9) in mind.

It is an electrifying time for stem cells. But we all need to avoid the trap of becoming so emotionally enamored with stem cells as medicines that we loosen our standards. We need to be patient enough to let researchers have the time to do their jobs in a structured, methodical and transparent way so that as soon as possible we will all benefit from the newest class of drugs that will reach the market to treat or prevent a whole host of medical conditions: stem cells.

If you feel that your disease has put you in a place for which patience is not an option, talk with your physician. Get second and maybe even third and fourth opinions before deciding whether or not to proceed. Reach out to stem cell scientists and the ISSCR as resources. Stem cells, when given in a reckless for-profit manner, by untrained physicians can indeed do more harm than good. When employed in a responsible manner backed by strong science, stem cells have a tremendous power for good. The key is specifically promoting the ethical use of stem cells as evidenced-based medicines not based on hype.

I do believe that stem cells are the next medical revolution on the horizon. In fact that revolution is already underway. I hope that through this book you now have a deeper understanding of stem cells and their potential clinical use. Stem cells are today's new frontier of medicine that will no doubt have an unimaginable impact on our lives, but even more so on the lives of many of our kids and grandchildren.

I find both joy and hope in the idea that stem cells have the potential to help our children and future generations avoid many of the serious health-related problems that we face today.

Index